My Life at the Wheel

Also by Lynne Sharon Schwartz

Fiction
Two-Part Inventions
The Writing on the Wall
Referred Pain (stories)
In the Family Way
The Fatigue Artist
Leaving Brooklyn
Disturbances in the Field
The Melting Pot and Other Subversive Stories
Acquainted with the Night (stories)
Balancing Acts
Rough Strife
Truthtelling

Nonfiction
This Is Where We Came In
Not Now, Voyager
Ruined by Reading
Face to Face
We Are Talking About Homes
A Lynne Sharon Schwartz Reader

Poetry
No Way Out But Through
See You in the Dark
In Solitary

For Children
The Four Questions

My Life at the Wheel

For information, address DELPHINIUM BOOKS, INC.,
16350 Ventura Boulevard, Suite D
PO Box 803
Encino, CA 91436

Library of Congress Cataloguing-in-Publication Data is
available on request.
ISBN 978-1-953002-31-0
23 24 25 26 27 LBC 5 4 3 2 1

Jacket and interior design by Colin Dockrill, AIGA

My Life at the Wheel

New and Selected Essays

Lynne Sharon Schwartz

Delphinium Books

CONTENTS

My Life at the Wheel.............................5

You Gotta Have Heart........................17

My Mother Speaks.............................59

The Renaissance.................................62

For My Father, Shaving......................67

Degrees of Separation.........................73

What I Don't Know............................76

The Other Henry James......................82

Trans Fish...93

Using a Cane.....................................97

First Loves..102

Beyond the Garden............................105

Only Connect.....................................110

"Give Me Your Tired, Your Poor . . .".........128

Time Off to Translate........................136

Detective Briscoe of the NYPD..........161

A Sort of Hero...................................164

Three Walks on Corn Hill Beach.........174

Introduction

I never thought seriously about writing a memoir, that is, the kind of narrative that would trace my life in a continuous line. I tend to see my past more as an assortment of segments, better suited for disguising into fiction, the form I've worked in most during my writing life. I did write two books considered memoirs, *Ruined by Reading* and *Not Now, Voyager*, but to my mind, they were less focused on personal history than on their subjects, reading and travel, as they impinged on my life. Lately, though, as these recent essays kept accumulating, some personal, some about books, some unclassifiable, I began to see that they were forming a collection of sorts. Something like a collage, where I could gather the pieces together and see what shape they might make. The prospect intrigued me, as collages have always intrigued me.

So I can safely say that the writings that follow are probably as close to an actual memoir as I'll ever get. Quite a few of the essays are about the process of becoming. As I read them over, I'm surprised that I appear more in a reactive than active mode, or mood. Becoming seems to occur in my response to events that insinuate themselves into my horizon and widen it. "Give Me Your Tired, Your Poor . . ." shows a young child's reaction to a puzzling, intimidating person; in "Degrees of Separation," again, as an adult I come to see what I couldn't know as a child; and in "You Gotta Have Heart" and "Using a Cane," I respond to situations unwanted but thrust on me.

Similarly, my troubled response to the events of September 11, 2001, is embedded in "Three Walks on Corn Hill Beach" and in "Harmony," near the end of the collection. Those two, and indeed most of the essays, were written a good while after the events that gave rise to them, specifically in the couple of years just before and after the arrival of the coronavirus in March 2020 (still not quite gone as I write). My reactions to that, like everyone's, have been complex and difficult, but I've had no urge to write about them. I've never managed to write about events right after they happen or in their midst. It can take a long time for my thoughts and words to assemble themselves, whether in essays or fiction. (I'd never make an efficient journalist.) Perhaps in a few years' time I'll be writing about the pandemic, whether it's over or—let's hope not—still going on.

I also felt a greater sense of authority writing about my parents, now long gone, as they appeared to me in my childhood, for instance in "For My Father, Shaving" or "The Renaissance." And at this distance I could write about my young self with a similar long-range perspective and irony.

Books have shaped me, perhaps even more than events, as I described in an earlier book, *Ruined by Reading.* Those who were avid child readers will understand what I mean. The novels of Henry James were powerful influences. James was the subject of my long-ago master's thesis, so it was striking to find, years later, an almost unknown novel of his, described in "The Other Henry James." And "Time Off to Translate" describes how I unexpectedly became a translator from Italian.

About the assorted shorter pieces, I can say only that, eccentric as they are, they nagged at my imagination, demanding to be written, like some minor itch or a craving for exotic food. "Beyond the Garden," originally a whimsical bit of fluff in response to a request by a long-gone feminist magazine, became more serious than I'd expected. "A Sort of Hero" came from a request by *The Review of Contemporary Fiction*, which was devoting an issue to the great Swiss modernist Robert Walser. I had nothing useful to add to the scholarly work that has accreted around Walser, but I had read his work so thoroughly and with such pleasure that I tried replicating his voice and his motifs. "A Refreshing Change Is in Your Future" describes, and presents, my untutored attempts to work in a new art form, not that the results remotely merit the label of "art." Instead of words, these concoctions were an early response to the shock and isolation of lockdown in the first months of the pandemic.

I have resisted the ever-present temptation to fictionalize, and done my best to stick to truth, both as a discipline and a debt owed to the past.

My Life at the Wheel

There is nothing so nice as being whisked somewhere in a car, very fast.

My father was to the motor born. He drove for pleasure when he was calm and drove for relief when he was enraged, and drove for the sake of driving. He'd take anyone anywhere; all you had to do was ask. "Come," he'd beckon when I was a child, "let's go for a ride." I'd hop in and we were off. No seat belts to fuss with back then.

He drove rashly and aggressively but with perfect control, and I always felt quite safe as well as excited to be his passenger. Excited because, beyond the eccentricities of his moves—cutting across lanes of traffic to make a turn, or driving in lanes blocked off for construction—we were playing the game of life: driving was triumphing over others, getting there not only quicker, but with panache. His driving was a performance: he wanted to steal the show. Buses, other cars, pedestrians, even street furniture like lampposts or mailboxes were impediments to his progress. He would keep up a running commentary on his fellow drivers, a commentary rich with derision. Anything moving less nimbly than we seemed too risible to exist, never mind occupy the road. He had no major accidents and just a few minor ones, David-and-Goliath fender benders, born of hubris.

This all held me spellbound. I assumed driving skill was an inherited trait and I would become the same kind of bold, virtuoso driver as my father. This, alas, did not happen. Quite the contrary. Perhaps because, unlike my brother and sister, I didn't have the benefit of my father's instruction but learned at a driving school in Boston, a city known for its fearsome traffic.

My brother was born with driving in his DNA: from the age of two he could identify the make and name of any car pictured in a glossy magazine, and grew up to be as gifted at the wheel as our father, though less wedded to the performance aspect. My sister learned to drive under my father's harrowing tutelage. He would have her maneuver through heavily congested lower Manhattan while he dashed in and out of the car on business errands or for quick phone calls. "Drive around the block if you see a police car," and if she demurred, "What could happen?" he would say. She turned out a good driver too, an easygoing, reliable driver, I don't know how.

I heard a neighbor casually remark that whenever you step into a car, you're taking your life in your hands. Certain words stick in the mind, or the mind clings to them. This bit of warped wisdom wasn't even true, or true only in the sense that any venture out of bed might be life-threatening. But I never forgot it. As a driver, I was alarmed by the other cars whizzing past. I was less afraid of being killed than of killing someone. Failing that, I would do something clumsy and gauche and be mocked for it, as my father had mocked other drivers: I thoughtlessly assumed everyone must harbor the same antagonism as he did. My fear was a species of social anxiety, the anxiety of an inexperienced person at a formal event, like meeting royalty, afraid of committing a ghastly blunder.

The road had its grown-up male rites, the ignorance of which could bring lasting shame: how to merge, how to get gas, how to rent a car, and Heaven forbid, how to fix a flat tire. What's a girl like me doing in charge of this powerful machine about whose workings I understood nothing? Even the radio was a challenge, never mind the more intricate parts. I dreaded a minor accident more than a major one. In the latter case I'd be unconscious or dead and the police would take care of everything.

At the same time I felt the opposite, a dread of my own power: I sensed that I could be a bold driver. My father's driving genes, lurking within, might suddenly assert themselves. I could be a master of the road. I yearned for this and dreaded it. The dread was strongest when I was alone. With passengers aboard I was calm: surely I wouldn't risk anyone's life by letting those anarchic genes run rampant. I was most at ease driving with my children—I would never endanger them. In their presence I was unquestionably a grown-up, entitled to the driver's seat.

The first car of my adult life was a red Renault Dauphine my husband and I named Dauphie. A babyish name; we were hardly more than babies ourselves, recently married at an absurdly young age, going to graduate school. Joining us in our quest for adventure, Dauphie traveled across the Atlantic to Italy in the bottom of a ship called the *Leonardo da Vinci*, probably in more comfortable circumstances than ours in a tiny room up above. It was a long trip during which we played deck tennis and ate more meals each day than one usually does. We were relieved to dock at Naples and begin the perilous and splendid drive along the Amalfi coast to our destination, Rome. We drove Dauphie all around Rome and to many small cities in Italy and grew fond of her.

But her behavior changed when we returned to the States. Parts began falling off, such as an inner door handle, the rearview and side-view mirrors, which we reattached with duct tape. It was as if she were protesting being back in the States after having seen so many new and thrilling places in Italy. Also perhaps she had enjoyed being close to the place of her birth, France. Indeed she went through France on the way from Rome to Amsterdam, where we boarded a ship home called the *Rotterdam* and again ate far more often than necessary.

The worst symptom Dauphie developed on returning home was a refusal to move in reverse. This made parking difficult on the hilly streets of Boston's Beacon Hill, where we had found our first real jobs. When we stopped to pay a toll and overshot the booth (this was before EZ-Pass), whoever was driving had to step out of the car to reach the toll taker's outstretched hand. We lost our affection for Dauphie. She would have to be replaced.

But we couldn't afford a new car or even a used one, and Dauphie, with her idiosyncrasies and decorative patches of duct tape, would not be worth much in a trade. Fortunately my mother was ready to get rid of her car so she offered it to us.

A word here about my mother's driving history: My mother learned to drive in her fifties, when she and my father moved from Brooklyn to the nearby suburbs, where you must drive in order to have a life. Before that, he did all the driving, even taking her to visit her mother in Williamsburg every Saturday afternoon. He would have a haircut at his favorite barbershop in the neighborhood while she and I spent the afternoon sitting around the kitchen table with her mother and her three sisters, recounting the week's gossip, shelling walnuts and drinking glasses of tea.

Given their very different temperaments, my parents knew it would never do for him to teach her, as he had done successfully with my brother and sister. She took lessons and eventually passed the test. She was plucky and confident, a confidence quite misplaced, since her driving was the stuff of farce. For a good while into her driving career she believed the rearview mirror was for powdering her nose. When first driving on the Palisades Parkway, she was astonished by the friendliness of her new neighbors—all the other drivers were waving at her. Finally it dawned on her that she was going north in the southbound lanes.

Once a week she came into Manhattan, our next home, to take care of my small children so I could get to my part-time job. She said, "I always thought a woman should stay home with her children, but in your case I see you can't. So I'm coming." On one occasion she called to explain her lateness: she'd inexplicably missed the proper downtown exit and had driven from one river of Manhattan to the other, ending up in Queens because she couldn't find a place to make a left turn. None of this daunted her. She had an enviable devil-may-care attitude to driving, perhaps from decades of being my father's passenger.

My mother's hand-me-down was a shiny gold-colored Mercury and much larger than we were accustomed to. We accepted the old car gratefully and called it Sarah, in honor of my mother. The car was similar to her in its shininess and boldness; it was oversized like my mother, and like her, it behaved generously to us. Friends teased us for having such a large, flamboyant car—it was the era of rebellion in the sixties and we scorned symbols of middle-class materialism—but nonetheless we loved Sarah because she was willing and cooperative and didn't exhibit any of the neurotic and disabling symptoms of her more exotic predecessor.

I drove Sarah when it was unavoidable. I was assured that were I to drive regularly, I would eventually feel at ease. Yet the idea of getting behind the wheel filled me with dread.

I tried to adopt my father's outlook: What could happen? Plenty. The steering wheel could lock in place and the car could run amok. The gas pedal could get stuck, or maybe the brake: one way or another, I would be unable to stop. Should I drive until I ran out of gas? That might take me to Canada or beyond.

Despite all of this nonsense, I did like the feeling of unlocking the car and climbing in, breezy and grown up, looking like any ordinary driver, not someone who was taking her life in her hands. But the cloud of dread shadowed me. I planned each trip in detail, reviewing every turn, every traffic light, every lane change. Once I started the engine, the cloud would disperse. What a relief to be driving and not anticipating driving! Anticipation is almost always worse than whatever is anticipated. In fact, I handled the car well enough; I liked to drive fast, and at times I even felt the elation of power, of controlling this menacing and mysterious machine. I even got in the habit of cursing other drivers, as my father did, but more for the ritual, without any passionate conviction.

The only time I could truly relax behind the wheel was the year I spent in Hawaii, where I drove to work in Honolulu three days a week on a spectacular highway that wound through towering green mountains scored by ancient volcanos, as if a giant had scraped the hills with his sharp fingernails. The drivers in Hawaii were disarmingly courteous. There was none of the competitive spirit one finds on the mainland; road rage seemed unimaginable. In Hawaii, drivers slow down to allow you to merge, one of the moves I found scariest. My instinct was to close my eyes and dash into the traffic, hoping for the best. But Hawaiian drivers slow down and wave you on with a special hand gesture out the window, making a fist with the thumb up and turning the hand from left to right. So driving there was almost pleasant.

I don't remember Sarah's end, but I imagine she succumbed to the natural infirmities of age, like her namesake. As it happened, around the time Sarah expired, my sister and brother-in-law were about to trade in their old car and they offered it to us instead.

This car was also large but not as large as Sarah, and it was the opposite of shiny—a sort of nondescript gray-green color—and it was generally self-effacing and dull in every way. Self-effacing in the sense that if you forgot where you parked it in a large lot, you might pass by several times before you recognized it. Because of its flagrant dullness, we called the car Herman, and before long came to feel affection for him.

Despite Herman's mild nature, he did manage to get into trouble. My husband had begun his graduate studies in Philadelphia and the dean of his department hosted a welcome party for students in his manorial suburban house. When we arrived, a good many cars were already crammed in the driveway and on the surrounding lawn. We finally inched into a space behind a classy MG sports car and joined the party. Later, retrieving Herman, we found he had inadvertently locked bumpers with the low-slung sports car. An offense so unlike harmless Herman, made more distressing when we learned that the car trapped beneath ours belonged to our host, the dean, who could not hide his dismay. It was not an auspicious beginning to Harry's graduate studies. Several of the male students came out to help lift Herman off the MG. The incident haunted us. Over the next two years, whenever we encountered the dean at a social event, we felt awkward and wanted to flee.

Back again in New York City, Herman was stolen. It was

an era of car thefts in our neighborhood. Some thieves didn't even bother with subterfuge. Our niece from Long Island had come to live with us while she attended college. Her first night in our apartment, rather late, I found her staring out the window. When I inquired, she said she saw someone use tools to open the door of a car parked just below our window and, after some effort, got it started and drove off. I explained that she had witnessed a car theft and must call the police should it happen again. Although everyone knew that by the time the police arrived, any stolen car would be far away.

We were sorry to lose Herman, and to lose him in such a sordid way—an unworthy end to a respectable career. But one must move on. At this point we could afford to buy our own car, and we chose a red Toyota station wagon. Our children were now old enough to take part in the naming of the car, its christening. We were all fans of the TV show *The Electric Company*, for kids who had graduated from *Sesame Street*, and which featured the entrancing voice of Morgan Freeman, soon to become a star. We loved an absurd, zen-like episode titled "Love of Chair," in which a man simply sat in a chair. It ended with the out-of-nowhere question "And what about Naomi?"—at which we burst out laughing. So we agreed to name the Toyota Naomi.

Naomi remained with us for many years and made many trips. She was a good-natured car but whimsical. Like the original Dauphie, parts of her had a tendency to fall off. Also, she was accident prone. Not serious accidents; rather, she was the victim of more aggressive vehicles. Often we would find her injured. She had dents and scrapes all over, like a boy who's been in a fight. We covered her injuries with duct tape, the automotive Band-Aid, and in time she had so many stripes that she resembled a racing car. Which was ironic, because one of her whimsical traits was a refusal to accelerate quickly.

Parking spaces in New York City were scarce and coveted. A friend of mine claimed she could tell when people on the street were heading to their cars, i.e., to vacate a space. It was something about their purposeful gait, or perhaps their hands in their pockets, already fingering their keys. So she lurked nearby and followed them, usually meeting with success.

To make matters worse, during that period in civic life, cars had to be moved from one side of the street to the other several times a week for street cleaning. If you didn't get out early, the spaces would all be taken. Harry, who was then working from home, hated stopping precisely at noon to move Naomi, then sitting in her until the street cleaning truck lumbered past. Many of our neighbors were doing the same thing, so the ritual became a social occasion as well as a competitive sport. I liked gazing down from our third-floor window as drivers struggled to fit into tiny spaces.

Once I started working at home, it was only fair that I share the burden. Unlike driving, it didn't frighten me since all it entailed was pulling out of the parking space, making a U-turn, then finding a spot across the street. Because I parked so much more often than I actually drove, I became an excellent parker, something of which I was proud. I still am, even though we no longer own a car.

Over the years I've shared the driving halfway across the country; I've driven through rain and sleet and hail and dark of night, on dirt roads and bracing freeways. I've learned to live with my dread, as one accommodates more serious dreads. A police car rolling into view means they're coming to get me for some foolish infraction. The threatening blare of a horn means I've been clumsy and given offense. "Ask not for whom the bell tolls . . ."

There came a time when Naomi was too debilitated to drive anymore. Our children were nearly grown and could navigate the city on their own. Our parents were gone so there was no need to visit them. The only thing was, how to get rid of her. Like Dauphie, she was too moribund to be traded in. My husband worked frequently in New Jersey and he decided to abandon her there, heartless as that seemed after her years of service. One night he removed everything that might serve as identification, left her in a parking lot in a Jersey town just over the George Washington Bridge, and took a bus home. We were free of her! No more car to move, no more rolls of duct tape to buy. Imagine our surprise when a couple of weeks later we got a phone call from a police officer in New Jersey. He announced that he had good news. I'm happy to tell you, sir, that we've found your car, he said. You can come and pick it up. He reasonably assumed it had been stolen. Apparently an envelope with Harry's name and address had been found under one of the seats.

It is illegal to abandon cars. Harry tried to match the officer's enthusiasm. Oh, thank you so much, he said. I'll come right over.

So we had Naomi back. We drove her around for a while longer, until a man working in a nearby service station said he could fix her up and use her. He offered fifty dollars, a generous sum, considering her condition. Though she might have been sporting fifty dollars' worth of duct tape.

I was relieved, thinking I need never drive again. In that mood of relief, I spoke to my older sister about my driving anxieties. I thought she might understand, having grown up with and been taught to drive by our father. She was sympathetic, but dismissed my father's approach: "He was a madman on the road. You can't let his driving influence you." She said I had the right to drive in whatever manner felt comfortable. The car was simply a means of getting somewhere. She had no contempt for other drivers; she had no interest at all in other drivers. The road was a community in which we all pursued our destination at our own pace. Naturally we observed the social contract, for our common good. But essentially we were following our individual paths. A new slant on the game of life on the road.

You might think that after this great yet banal revelation, I would drive with ease. But that did not happen. To my father, and to me, when I was his passenger, the road was not a cooperative community but the state of nature. And the allure of that state was powerful. To move with such arrogance and abandonment, such predatory skill! But I didn't yield to the lure, and surely it was better so.

Better because we were not yet finished with cars. We were so used to having a car around, like a family member. . . . We bought a used car. At that time the family was hooked on the weekly TV episodes of John Galsworthy's *The Forsyte Saga*. Our kids loved to act out the moment, in an art gallery, when charming and flirtatious Fleur Forsyte deliberately drops her handkerchief, and the man she has designs on retrieves it. "FF. Fleur Forsyte," she trills with mock surprise. "That must be me." Inevitably, our next car was named Fleur.

Soon our children were grown and gone, with lives of their own. Fleur wore out quickly, as such coquettes often do. We replaced her with a used car, so nondescript that I barely remember it. We were past fifty: our childish habit of naming and personifying cars was over, a sobering sign of maturity. When I drove this nameless car, I tried to remember my sister's wise advice about the road of life. I muttered curses when a nearby driver did something clumsy or inept. Aside from that harmless indulgence, I observed the social contract, but I longed to be in a state of nature. The tension was exciting. Anything might happen. Elation, power, and dread swirled in my every cell.

Our daughter and son-in-law were in the habit of borrowing this unloved car for weekend trips, and one Sunday they called to say it had been in an accident on the way home. Nothing serious; they were unhurt. Our son-in-law, an experienced driver from Minnesota, where kids often learn to drive around twelve years old, had been going 15 miles an hour on an exit ramp when our car and another attempted to occupy the same space. The car was only slightly banged up, but the insurance company pronounced it dead and refused any compensation.

I didn't care anything about the car; I was ready to live without it. My husband wasn't too upset either: he had recently announced that after this car died he never wanted to own another car again. Enough! What we cared about was our daughter, who was in the early stages of pregnancy. But we were assured that the impact was not enough to shake anything up.

Several months later our granddaughter was born in perfect condition, and while we never had another car again, we had a new member of our family who could do so many wonderful things a car could not, and instead of causing dread brought pure delight.

You Gotta Have Heart

Cigarettes

A pack of Vantage containing two cigarettes was in my coat pocket when I arrived at the hospital. It was a bitter morning in late December. The angiogram was scheduled for eleven o'clock, at least I had been told to be there at eleven o'clock, but it didn't take place until three in the afternoon. I made a scene over this at hourly intervals, first arguing with the receptionist in the waiting room, then insisting on being admitted past the swinging double doors behind which others before me had disappeared, to confront whoever was in charge back there. Just because they were the authorities, the medical bureaucracy, I wasn't going to be a meek cipher in their hands. I would begin this journey in the right spirit.

But no matter how vehemently I railed against the injustice and lack of consideration, the angiogram didn't take place until three o'clock.

I was in the hospital for the replacement of an aortic valve, what the surgeon afterward—while I was still unconscious—told my family was a "very nasty" valve. He had advised that I stay at the hospital after the angiogram, since the surgery would begin around six the next morning: why go home merely to get up in the middle of the night to return? This seemed sensible and I agreed. My plan was that once the angiogram was over—I understood you had to lie still for an hour or so afterward—assuming I survived, I would go out with my husband for a cup of coffee and smoke what would be my last cigarettes for quite a while. Maybe forever. Again, assuming I survived. Whenever doctors or nurses lean over my body preparing to insert something in a place not designed to be penetrated, I feel endangered. During the angiogram they would be making a hole in my groin and threading a tube straight up to my heart; it sounded like an unwieldy as well as unnatural procedure, but many before me had survived it and most likely I would too.

While it was in progress, though, I had my doubts. I wasn't completely unconscious; I had enough awareness to hear the older doctor telling the younger one—a very young doctor; his bare face sticking out of the plastic shower cap was cherubic—what to do, how to guide the tube inside me and so on. I said, "Why so much instruction? Are you actually teaching him how to do this on me?" The older doctor laughed, ha ha. "No, of course he knows how to do it."

I didn't want to distract them from the lesson, and so I desisted. Also, I really wasn't up for a dialogue; I was too entranced by the drug. I'm not sure what they gave me—if I were, I'd try to get a prescription—but it was something that leaves you half awake and aware, and yet everything happening to your body, as well as to the people working on it, seems at a great remove. So close and yet so far. Something unnatural is happening to you, but it's painless, and anyway, "you" are not the same singular entity as before: there's the body that belongs to you (who else?) and then there's your dimmed consciousness, looking on from afar. A great drug, but it wears off quickly.

Instead of carrying out my plan of the cup of coffee and cigarette afterward, I found myself being led into an elevator by an orderly, brought to an upper floor and assigned a room, a rather nice private room: a luxury floor. The room had the usual hospital paraphernalia and TV protruding from the wall like a hunter's stuffed moose head, but it also had the mildly pleasant, expectant scentless air of a hotel room, and that was how I intended to treat it. I began getting out of the grotesque hospital gown—white with little blue circles, not dots but donut-like circles, little *O*'s. Later I found that this garment, whose only accommodations to the shape of the human body were enormous sleeves and a string to be tied at the neck, also came in sky blue with no circles.

I can't help wondering if there is some reason—economy, perhaps, or mere thoughtlessness?—why these hospital gowns have to be quite so humiliatingly ugly. I know they have to be open so that the body within is fully accessible to the professionals who will handle it, but must it be ugly besides? Adding insult to injury, so to speak? Would it cost so much more to use the services of a designer, maybe not someone first-rate like Donna Karan or Ralph Lauren, that would be an extravagance, but some young person just starting out who'd be grateful for the work? It would be only a one-time thing.

I was reaching for my street clothes when a nurse came into the room. "What are you doing?" she asked, gazing at me and my husband, who sat in one of the pink plastic chairs.

"Getting dressed," I said.

"You're supposed to leave the gown on," she said.

"My surgery isn't until tomorrow morning and it's not even six yet. We're going out to get a cup of coffee." Despite my pose of bravado, I knew enough not to mention the cigarettes.

She was no Sue Barton but a stern-looking nurse of the old school: stocky, short hair in a mannish cut, sharp voice, no nonsense. "You're not going anywhere. This is your room. You'll stay here until they call for you."

"I beg your pardon," I said. "The surgery isn't until tomorrow, as I said. The angiogram is over. There's nothing you need me for. I'm going out. I promise I'll return for dinner," I said with a little chuckle, to lighten the situation. I didn't want to make this a fight over my civil rights, or rather I did—but without being pompous, as such fights are liable to be. I tied my sneakers as I spoke.

"You don't understand," she said, a bit more gently, as if indeed the rules hadn't been explained to me properly. "You are a patient."

My mother used to tell me that I had no patience. She also used to say, during my minor childhood illnesses, that I was a terrible patient, I suppose meaning fretful, demanding and impatient. Maybe because I've been labeled as impatient, I've always disliked the homophonic connection between the noun "patient," the sick person, and the adjective "patient," the character trait. They come from the same Latin root meaning suffering or enduring, and it's easy to see why that root branched out in the two directions and parts of speech. But that doesn't mean that a patient necessarily is or ought to be patient, that is to say, according to the dictionary definition, "enduring pain, trouble, affliction, hardship, etc., with fortitude, calmness, or quiet submission." Certainly it makes practical sense to endure one's ailment with fortitude and calmness (not that practical sense ever played a large part in determining my attitudes). But must a patient also endure with "quiet submission" the thousand and one well-documented indignities of hospital life? I would think a patient's patience is already being sufficiently tried by illness; she shouldn't be expected to muster still more reserves of patience for those indignities. Rather it's the doctors and nurses who should be patient with the already patient patient.

All the same, after my husband went home and I began anticipating the events of the next morning, the fighting spirit deserted me. I was a patient. I put on the hospital gown, ate the hospital dinner, and settled into bed with a fat Henning Mankell mystery. All that was missing was a cigarette, one of the two in my coat pocket, but I didn't dare. It was a good thing I didn't, because the nurse entered and seemed pleased to find I had surrendered like a chastised child. She gave me a stack of papers to sign granting the hospital permission to do with me as they would, and I signed without really reading them, just a quick glance. I was in no mood to contemplate whatever I was agreeing to. Then she gave me a fat folder full of information about hearts and heart surgery, complete with diagrams and charts. "This literature may be helpful to you," she said. "It will familiarize you with your surgery, and with what goes on in the heart in general, how it functions and how to take good care of it."

I accepted the folder politely but had no intention of spending what might be my final hours reading its contents. In my heart I was thinking, So this "literature" will tell me what goes on in the heart? As if I didn't know! I'd spent years of my life reading about the heart. There was little I didn't know. *The Heart Is a Lonely Hunter. The Heart of the Matter. The Heart of Matter. In the Heart of the Country. In the Heart of the Heart of the Country. A Simple Heart. Near to the Wild Heart. The Mortgaged Heart. Heart of Darkness. Change of Heart. Crimes of the Heart. Habits of the Heart.* The heart has its reasons, Pascal said.

The Surgeon

Weeks before the surgery, I met the surgeon for the first time. He was a young man, quite good-looking in the com-

mon way of well-bred American white males, so common I
barely notice them: dark hair, squarish face, neatly shaped
features. Charlie Sheen, say, or a less charismatic Tom Cruise.
Courteous manners. He explained the "procedure." I asked
him what kind of valve, animal or artificial, he would use
to replace my faulty one. I thought I'd have some say in the
choice once I was apprised of the advantages and disadvan-
tages of each, but now that we sit here contemplating the surgery, I realize he's not the kind of doctor who will welcome
my input; he is most definitely the decider, as George Bush
used to say, and that's okay with me because I don't really
have an opinion. He says animal.

"What kind of animal? A pig?"

"No. A horse."

There is a pause, as I consider horses as opposed to pigs.
"This may sound like a silly question," I say, "but isn't a horse
valve a little large for me?"

He laughs. I made him laugh, quite unintentionally.
There was a saying we had back in Brooklyn, that some girls
think they're hot shit because they can make a man laugh in
bed, the joke being that this is pretty easy to do, within the
range of almost anyone. "We don't use the entire valve," he
says. "We make a valve from material in the horse's heart."

Oh. What about those horses? Is it like organ trans-
plants—someone young and healthy is in an auto accident
and their intact, barely used organs are rushed to a patient
who needs them? No, I doubt it. Horses don't get into auto
accidents. Are they horses who've outlived their usefulness
and are put out to pasture, like Black Beauty, whom I wept
over in adolescence, to spend the remainder of their lives at
ease, as in a nursing home? (Though people in nursing homes
tend to decline and die faster than those cared for at home.)
And then the horses die of natural causes but have agreed

beforehand to allow their organs to be used for humanitarian purposes? I mean, of course, that their owners agreed. Perhaps their owners got paid for the heart parts; yes, surely they got paid.

Now that I think of it, sitting here facing the young, generically handsome and self-assured doctor, I actually prefer a horse to a pig, if I have to have some other species inside me. I don't feel fastidious or repelled by the prospect of carrying around a part from another species; after all, we're all in this together, all creatures great and small. Nor am I a snob about animals. But I think most people would allow that horses are more attractive than pigs. As I'm staring at the doctor—a button on his right shirt cuff is loose and dangling; it could fall off any minute—it occurs to me that perhaps Orthodox Jews with a faulty aortic valve would not permit a pig's valve to be lodged inside them. If their doctor opted for a pig, they might protest and insist on a horse—no cloven foot. If no horses were available, those people would have to have an artificial valve. Also I read somewhere that Orthodox Jews, whose wives and daughters wear wigs covering their natural hair, stopped permitting wigs made of Indian hair. Indian hair is the best hair for wigs, and perhaps the best hair all around, period. There is a thriving business in selling Indian women's hair. But the Orthodox Jews thought that some of the original women's Hindu-ness might have infiltrated into the hair and thus would violate the heads of their new wearers. Well, I'm not an Orthodox Jew so I needn't concern myself with hair just now, or with the doctor's loose button. Just pigs and horses.

Like a pubescent girl, I love horses. I even rode horses, though not well, in my teen years. My family spent the summers in a bungalow colony in the Catskills whose aggressive dullness I loathed, but its saving grace was the nearby hotel where you could rent horses and ride around on the dirt roads. My favorite horse was called Brownie, very gentle, and I learned to trot, to post properly, and even to canter, before I got old enough to stay home alone in the summers. In Brooklyn a few times I rented horses at a stable near Bergen Beach and rode along the ocean. I felt I was in a movie: the surf, the sand, the sky, the horse and me on it. I rode just two or three more times as an adult, and then the equestrienne part of my life was over.

But I do know horses, at least a bit, and I would like to know the provenance of the piece of horse heart about to be lodged in my own: was he or she a farm horse, a police horse, maybe a prize race horse? I enjoy the races. I've been to the track lots of times, both Belmont and Saratoga, with my husband and friends: could I possibly be harboring a piece of a horse I've seen in a race, a horse I might have bet on, and won with?

"Okay," I said. "A horse." I tried to think of suitable and intelligent questions to ask. "How do you get to the valve? I mean mine, not the horse's."

"We reach in," he said, not exactly tersely, but in a tone that meant he didn't care to elaborate.

We reach in. I've remembered those words ever since as a kind of magic formula, an open sesame, as it were. So ominous, so graphic and yet so vague, enigmatic. They reach into me. Me! This man would touch my heart as no man ever had before.

The only other question I had for the surgeon was, Will I die by your knife? And it certainly wasn't suitable to ask that. What did I expect? Of course he would say I'd be fine. He'd probably say, with a confident chuckle, that he'd done this hundreds of times, thousands. Later on I thought of many specific and important questions, but at the time, confronting him before the surgery, my mind was blank. It seemed I should know him better than one brief appointment's worth, since he would be opening my chest and handling my heart. And yet he was a virtual stranger. It was like going to bed with someone when all you know about him is his name, if that.

"How long is the recovery period?" I asked as I stood up to leave.

"Two weeks," he said.

Mild, Moderate, Severe, Critical

It wasn't as if I was undertaking this surgery under duress, as it may appear from my recalcitrance. No, strictly speaking, I chose it. I'd known about the faulty valve for several years, but at first the cardiologist, a gentle, rotund, clear-eyed youngish man, said the situation was "mild." Unless and until it progressed through "moderate" to "severe," to "critical," at which point it would require surgery, I should forget about it and carry on my normal life. In that instance I was more than willing to obey the doctor without question. At this rate, "critical" would not arrive for many years, I thought, maybe so many years that I would already be dead and therefore no surgery would be necessary. I carried on. Until one day after a stress test, the cardiologist directed his steady gaze at me and said the state of the valve had passed "severe" and was near "critical." He strongly recommended surgery. Soon.

"Are you serious?" I said, still panting from the stress test, sitting on the examining table, my legs dangling down. The idea of me undergoing surgery had no reality for me, even though I'd seen several members of my family go through it. From my husband's bypass operation six years ago, I knew intimately what open heart surgery entailed.

"Very serious. If you don't do it, you have a fifty-fifty chance of dying of this in two years."

Aha. Something clicked in my mind as I quickly moved into rebuttal mode. "But that means I also have a fifty-fifty chance of living. So . . ." I shrugged.

"Okay then," he said, his kindly face unchanged. I guess he'd heard every kind of response, even flippant. "Make it four years. Then your chances of dying really improve."

The doctors, I later learned, call invasive surgery an insult. (My husband's doctor referred to his heart surgery as "the second insult." When I asked what was the first, he said, "Birth.") Now I could see the aptness of the term. More than repelled and frightened by the prospect of surgery, I also felt insulted—in advance—especially as I recalled the array of side effects my husband, sister and brother had experienced. But I didn't want to die in two years, or even four. So I chose to be a patient instead.

The Dead

In the two years just before my surgery, two of my closest friends died. They both lived right nearby, Glenda around the corner for twenty years and Rebecca about three blocks west for even longer. Glenda died of a brain tumor, or perhaps it was ovarian cancer that spread to her brain. She died in Australia, where she was born, so I didn't see her in the last few months, only spoke to her on the phone. By the end her voice on the phone sounded like static. Rebecca died of lung cancer. I saw her a lot during that illness, except near the very end when I called to ask if I could come over and she said, "I love you, dear, but I can't see you." I always was touched when she called me dear. I don't find it easy to use endearments, except to children. Of course this time my pleasure was marred by disappointment and grief.

We were all writers together. I met Rebecca at Yaddo, an artists' colony, and though I felt slightly intimidated by her—she was very shy, I later learned, and this gave her an air of aloofness—I invited her to take a walk one afternoon. Yaddo is in Saratoga Springs, where the famous horse races take place, and on our walk through a back lane we passed stables and horses meandering around a meadow, a tranquil scene. Little did I know then, thirty-two years earlier, that one day a piece of horse would prolong my life, though not any of the horses we saw that day—they don't live that long.

After that walk we were good friends for thirty-one years. I met Glenda because I reviewed a book of hers for *Ms.* magazine. The book, full of bizarre and darkly whimsical happenings, intrigued me; I thought the person who wrote it must be odd and eccentric, and so I went to a reading she gave in an East Side bookstore to check her out. I was hesitant about introducing myself to the author of a book—I hadn't published any books at the time, only short pieces in magazines—but she was approachable and grateful for my review. We discovered that we were neighbors and we, too, became friends for decades.

I introduced the two of them, and we formed a kind of trio, meeting in the late afternoon in the West End Bar near Columbia University to drink and smoke and talk about our work and about life. We had met as writers and continued that way, although as our lives became enmeshed and our children grew up, we talked about everything else under the sun. We were very different but we came to understand one another perfectly because we were intuitive about reading character, the signs of character. Glenda, who was not odd or eccentric in any immediately obvious way, had her Australian accent and spoke in a soft, gentle voice and had impeccable manners, and in that soft gentle voice she said outrageous and radical things. Rebecca was older and seemed to carry the wisdom of the ages in her head capped by sleek auburn hair shaped like a bowl, but she carried her burden lightly, with wit; she was from Georgia and had a pronounced Southern drawl and a wry skepticism about most things, but a sentimental streak that came out in her love of cats and dogs. There was a spell when I would ride my bike down Riverside Drive first thing in the morning, and I often met Rebecca walking her dog, who she insisted had said a few words and even shed a few tears. Glenda drove a large car and I'd sometimes meet her going to move her car in accordance with the parking regulations, as one must do on the Manhattan streets, using her talent of spotting people about to vacate their spaces.

Sometimes two of us would meet, and I wondered about the combinations of two out of three: for instance, how the two of them sounded and spoke when I wasn't present. The ways I spoke with each of them alone were very different; this was inevitable, given how unlike we were. We resembled three interlocking circles—I'm thinking of the old Ballantine Ale logo, the three circles standing for Ballantine's salient qualities, purity, body and flavor. None of us represented any of those qualities especially, but the design fit. We shared a considerable common area yet each of us had a large private space of our own.

Anyway, they died, Glenda in 2007 and Rebecca in 2008 and I was bereft. After Glenda died so far away, Rebecca and I felt the lack. Even though our friendship was rich on its own, we would never again know that special interlocking threesome. Then Rebecca got sick, and though we never said it aloud, we both knew I would continue with a double loss, missing the particular quality of our friendship, in which we could say anything that occurred to us and neither of us would ever be shocked, and sometimes we need not even say it—a meaningful look could convey volumes. Rebecca was unshockable and through her I learned to be the same.

So when I went for my heart surgery, I thought: I am the last of the three, and maybe this year, the third year, 2009, will be my turn. As they wheeled me into the operating room, before the anesthetic that put me out, I had a glimpse of them in an afterlife that resembled the old West End Bar, where we used to meet in the ancient booths, dark and smoky, nursing our drinks of choice: wine, bourbon, and for me, Diet Pepsi; I was never much of a drinker. They're chatting away. I don't know what the two of them sound like alone, without me, but I do manage to hear a few words in Glenda's gentle, now slightly anxious voice: "Where's Lynne? She's never this late." Then comes Rebecca's deep, bourbon-soaked drawl. "She'll turn up soon. She's very reliable that way."

Rehearsal

When I first came out of the operating room, I was adorned with lots of tubes, like someone who's just come from the Mardi Gras parade in New Orleans, bedecked with colorful necklaces and bracelets: tubes in several orifices and some where there were no orifices to begin with, such as the chest. Over the next few days the tubes were removed, one by one, some with a pop and some with a slither. My tubes were removed by a young Japanese physician's assistant named Elliot, a small doll-like man, delicate and slim as a miniature. I became fond of Elliot: something about his easygoing, competent manner combined with his delicate appearance inspired trust. He listened to my complaints with a benevolent neutrality, and often told me not to worry. Usually it's irritating to be told not to worry, but when Elliot said it, I didn't mind. He rarely smiled yet appeared serene, and he always explained exactly what he was about to do. With one of the tubes, a catheter, he said he would count, One, two, and then I must take a deep breath while he pulled it out, and that way it wouldn't hurt. One, two, breathe! Okay? I nodded. I breathed at the proper moment and it didn't hurt. Elliot praised me as if I were a kindergartner who had just written the letter *A* for the first time. I was proud of myself. It was a small accomplishment, true, but in my diminished condition, it was prideworthy. I felt so diminished and changed after the surgery that I couldn't take anything for granted anymore.

Pulling out the chest tube was more complicated as well as risky. It required some rehearsal. "We can't let any air get into the pleural cavity where this tube is," said Elliot, "so we have to practice first. You breathe, hold your breath, and I pull. Don't release your breath until I have the tube fully out. Do you understand?" I nodded.

"So we'll have a little rehearsal first," he said.

All this attention gave me a heady feeling, as if I had an important part in a play. As an adolescent I had aspired to be an actress and even studied acting for a while at the Henry Street Playhouse. One of my teachers was William Hickey, who later played, among other roles, a Mafia capo in a popular crime movie, a comedy. My aspirations came to nothing since I had little talent and much reserve. Still, with this in my past and diminished as I felt, the thought of a rehearsal of any kind brought a bit of excitement.

Elliot implied, or I inferred, that if air got into my pleural cavity, something terrible might happen to me. Surely less adept and alert people must have had this tube removed and

I'd never heard of any misfortunes resulting. And yet I felt it was a matter of life and death to do it right. "Breathe," said Elliot. "Hold. I pull." I held my breath while he pretended to pull. We rehearsed this two or three times.

"Okay, ready for the real thing?"

I was ready. Breathe, hold, pull. Together we did a perfect job. The final tube. I was on my own.

When he left, I had one of those marvelous epiphanies, like little mental orgasms, that unfortunately don't last long. If they did, we might never get back to the world's work. I was staring out at the Hudson River, wide, placid that day, steel gray in a wan sun, and suddenly I was seized by the glory, the miracle of being alive: I'd had that ghastly surgery and survived. It was done, I was blessed. None of the dailiness I'd fretted over before, family problems, work, dealings with banks and institutions, the construction across the street whose dumpsters' groans and beeps woke us at seven a.m., plus the dire state of the world, mattered any more. Compared to the wonder of life itself, those things were small and would sort themselves out. What mattered was that I would continue living. I didn't stop to think about in what condition I would live, too fine a point just then. Simply, as Strether in Henry James's novel *The Ambassadors* cries, "To live, to live!"

This feeling lasted, though not in the full intensity of its first strike, for about two and a half days. By the time I went home to start the labor of recovery, all the daily irritations came back and resumed their usual importance. And a little later on came the fear.

Recreation

Toward the end of my five-day sojourn in the hospital, when

I could walk around comfortably, I looked for entertainment other than staring out the window at the Hudson River from the pink plastic armchair in my room or reading my fat Henning Mankell mystery. I practiced going up and down stairs on the miniature wooden staircase near the nurses' station: it led nowhere, just five steps up and five down with a small platform on top. I made believe I was a political candidate about to deliver a campaign speech to an adoring crowd. I tried hanging out in the waiting room to feel part of the great outside, to hear conversations among civilians, not patients, conversations not about symptoms and procedures but about worldly things, sports, movies, traffic accidents, natural disasters . . .

A pretty fiftyish woman with lots of makeup and bright red hair elaborately carved into a tower-like pile asked me what I was "in for" and who was my surgeon. When I told her, she grew rhapsodic on the subject of my surgeon, a genius and savior. He had saved the lives of both her mother and her priest in conditions of extreme coronary drama. Furthermore, it had been he, she claimed, who operated so successfully a few years ago on former president Bill Clinton, although owing to hospital hierarchy and public relations, the feat had to be attributed to the head of the department.

What to say to this dubious bit of gossip? "You don't say," I said, using an expression from my childhood I believe I never used before.

The man next to her, whom I recognized as the husband of my new roommate—she had arrived attended by her family in the middle of the night—said, "I was in the living room and my wife was in the kitchen. I heard her calling, but to tell the truth, most of the conversation in the house is between my wife and the dog, so at first I assumed she was talking to the dog. What did that dog do now? But she kept calling so

I figured I better go see. She was lying on the floor groaning. When we got her here, we learned her aorta had ripped all the way down her body to her thigh." This sounded almost as gruesome as the murders Henning Mankell had concocted in his very long book.

It was, yet again, my surgeon who had saved her life. When she was brought to my room last night after the surgery, her appearance was not promising. She was quite overweight in her hospital gown, bedecked with tubes as I had been, and her skin was almost as gray as her long disheveled hair. She coughed all through the night, deep-wracking, wet, phlegmy coughs that seemed to rise from the pit of her stomach and spew upward like a geyser. At one point I rang for a nurse because the coughing alarmed me: she could die while I lay listening and then I would feel guilty for my inaction. The nurse came and murmured, "That's what happens when you have surgery after a lifetime of smoking."

That might have been me, I thought, given my lifetime of smoking, and I felt a moment of rare gratitude that it was not. Even though smoking wasn't the cause of my nasty valve, by rights I suppose I should have been coughing too. The woman's coughing reinforced the dogma that smoking has terrible effects. But it also suggested that in some cases it might not. I thought of the two cigarettes still in my coat pocket, in the closet of our hospital room. If my roommate weren't so sick, we could share them, have our last cigarette together, maybe in the bathroom with the door locked, like ten-year-olds.

The red-haired woman said, "I practically fell to my knees when I saw him after my mother came out of the recovery room. I didn't know how to thank him."

I hadn't seen the surgeon since my operation (he'd seen me but I was unconscious at the time) and hadn't given a thought to thanking him, which in retrospect feels ungrateful and ungracious. But at that point I was still thinking of him more as my assailant than my savior.

"So how did you thank him?" I asked.

"I'll give you a tip," she said, winking. "He likes Cabernet Sauvignon. By the case."

After a while I left the waiting room and took an exploratory walk down the corridors. I'd been encouraged to walk and for once was glad to follow orders. I like walking, even down a hospital corridor where you peek into rooms and see people in various states of disrepair and wearing charmless cotton gowns.

After my walk I returned to my chair at the picture window overlooking the Hudson and resumed the Henning Mankell mystery in which so many vile murders were described. I'm not an avid reader of mysteries; the only time I read them passionately was when I was around ten or twelve and gorged myself on Agatha Christie, Erle Stanley Gardner and *Ellery Queen's Mystery Magazine*. That quickly passed. But over the last few years I began listening to books on tape while I puttered and exercised in the morning, and found mysteries ideal for this purpose. Their merits aren't exclusively or primarily literary (although there are exceptions like P. D. James or Walter Mosley) so I needn't be afraid of missing some splendid phrase. The plots kept me going through the tedium of the exercises.

I discovered Henning Mankell on the shelves of a friend's guest room, where I stayed every Tuesday night one spring, when I taught a course at Bryn Mawr. This friend, with whom I'd gone to graduate school years earlier, had very exacting taste. She was so learned that for a long period she was head of the English Department at Bryn Mawr, so I assumed anything I found on her shelves would be high-class stuff. I started a Henning Mankell mystery one night and got so absorbed that I asked if I could borrow it for the train ride home and return it the following week.

Henning Mankell was Swedish and his detective, Kurt Wallander, lives in a small dismal town. He is depressed, like his town. He has lots of personal problems—his divorce; his relationships with his grown daughter and his aging father, an eccentric painter; his insomnia; and so on—besides the distressing murder cases assigned to him. He is often tired, cold, rain-soaked, and at odds with his fatuous supervisor. Wallander is an instinctive detective, thorough and painstaking rather than brilliant, and he quickly grew on me.

Mankell writes in short factual sentences that one by one are not striking, but when strung together become passages of vivid and forceful prose. Prose that's hard to stop reading. I kept the light on over my hospital bed each night, following the crimes and Wallander's team of eccentric detectives, the hunted and the hunters. The story was more grotesque than usual in a Mankell book, which is generally pretty grotesque. It involved a nurse seeking out and killing, in ingenious and sadistic ways, men who had abused and murdered women. Once she found them, she tied them up, placed them in sacks, starved them, and subjected them to other lengthy indignities I've managed to suppress. Reading about this treatment in the hospital after having my chest opened up, with people all around me whose chests had been opened up for one reason or another, felt satisfying. The world was full of atrocities, and the motives, benign or malignant, didn't seem to matter much. What mattered to me was simply the fact of the intrusions—that one person had performed them on a fellow human.

My attitude regarding the surgery was not the conventional, expected, or sensible one, that's for sure. It was more childish than adult. I knew that, and yet I clung to my resistance. It felt satisfying, far more so than quiet submission. Weeks after my release, when I met acquaintances or neighbors on the street and told them why they hadn't seen me around, some people responded by saying, Isn't it wonderful, the miracles they can perform these days! Aren't you lucky! and the like. I wanted to punch them. In some obscure nook of my brain I knew there was some truth to their words, but I wouldn't acknowledge that nook. There are times I still don't. It wasn't so much their actual words that disturbed me, but the gross ignorance behind them, ignorance of anything other than pure survival. Ignorance of what the newspapers call collateral damage. When listening to news reports of our current wars, I always find the collateral damage aspect the most intriguing. I wish the reporters would examine that damage further—who were these unintended victims whose lives end for no reason other than someone's faulty aim, or being in the wrong place at the wrong time? Why shouldn't their photos, with small intimate bios, appear on the back pages of the *New York Times*, as did those of the victims of the September 11 attacks?

Collateral damage as a result of surgery is quite different, of course. The patient is far from dead. Rather, the patient's entire body is analogous to the nation under siege, and regrettably, individual parts of the body unrelated to the main arena of attack are made to suffer.

The Hippocratic oath enjoins doctors to do no harm. But my surgery did harm; not only the sawing and hammering open of my chest and all that went with it, but the onslaught of fear—called depression by the professionals—that took me by surprise a couple of months later, and that allegedly strikes thirty to forty percent of heart surgery patients. So technically the doctors violated the oath. But of course they must, in order to do their work. Every painful treatment could be considered a violation of the oath. On the other hand, if my faulty valve caused my death within a couple of years (as the sweet-faced cardiologist predicted), and if the doctors had a remedy that could have averted that and yet they withheld it, that, too, would be doing harm. Arguably even more harm. You can't win: harm is done either way. Again, it's a matter of motives and results, means and ends, a slippery subject. Maybe the problem is with the oath itself, but of course no one would consider rescinding it, because who knows what doctors might do, left to their own devices.

With all this, our fate here in the hospital hinged on the doctors. We revered them and resented them, at least I did. I didn't resent them because they were helping me, as in, No good deed goes unpunished. No, I'd probably resent anyone I had to revere. Reverence is simply not part of my makeup. I dislike hierarchies, though I know they are ubiquitous in the animal kingdom. Long ago I worked for several years as a secretary for a Quaker organization and learned that Quakers don't use titles, even such common ones as Mr. and Mrs. (or now, Ms.). I was instructed, when I typed letters, to address the recipients, no matter how distinguished, by both names, e.g., Dear Albert Einstein, or Dear Nelson Mandela. Also, while the secretaries called each other and our own bosses by first names, we addressed all the other executives by their full names. I liked that. I still write letters that way. But I do call doctors Dr., despite the Quakers as well as feminism's eminently sensible policy: if the doctor calls you Lynne, you call him Joe. I don't want to get that chummy.

I shouldn't have been surprised that the people in the waiting room weren't discussing sports and earthquakes. They were relatives and friends of patients, and like those of us wearing the gowns, they were affected, or afflicted, by the hospital atmosphere, in which nothing is of any importance except living or dying. The awareness of the body's vulnerability, which normally doesn't need constant acknowledgment, is perpetual here. Anyone who finds himself in a hospital bed is by definition in danger. No wonder it's hard to focus on anything else.

At least that was so on the cardiac floor; maybe on less serious floors—broken bones, knee replacements, gallbladders—it's different. Here, we've come to be saved, to go on living. And we're rooting for each other, our sisters and brothers ambling through the halls dragging their IV poles, clinging to their slender dancing partner. There's a heartfelt camaraderie, a pure, unambiguous feeling you won't find in many other groups forced together by chance and circumstance. Most of us will probably live to go home—they certainly don't want us dying here—but how long after that?

"You Will Swallow the Tube"

Less than two weeks after the surgery, I find myself being prepared, in an extremely small room crowded with medical equipment, for a TEE, a transesophageal echocardiogram: a tube with a tiny camera at the end goes down the esophagus and behind the heart in order to see if there has been any stroke activity back there, any pieces—"grunge matter," one doctor called them—broken off during surgery that traveled to the brain. The TEE, one of several tests for stroke, is happening because a few days earlier, barely back home after my bonding with the anonymous horse, I looked down at the strips of tape bisecting my chest—some strips halfway off, some hanging longer than others, an ungainly tangle of tape—and asked why they were there. I never keep myself in such a messy state. My husband immediately realized, especially after a few more weird remarks, that something had gone wrong in my brain. Next stop, the emergency room of a nearby hospital, not the hospital where my "nasty valve" had been replaced.

I had either had a stroke or a TIA, a transient ischemic attack or mini-stroke. A TIA is better because it lasts only a short while and leaves no permanent neurological deficits. In my case, by the time we got to the ER, I had recovered and might have been better off going home.

The days were filled with tests or waiting for tests: they never took place exactly when scheduled. Some of the tests were very simple, such as the neurologist asking me to touch my nose then touch his finger, or to walk a straight line down the hospital corridor. Some were elaborate and involved sophisticated machinery, such as this upcoming TEE or yesterday's MRI. I tried to do well, as I had always tried on tests in school, even when there was nothing much I could do. Except during the MRI there were moments when the technician said, "Don't swallow now," and perversely, those were the moments when I felt the greatest need to swallow, and did. The heart has its reasons.

Some people can tolerate being slid into a tube like a roast going into the oven, followed by the sensation of being buried alive to the sound of jackhammers, and some can't. I assumed I'd be in the latter group, yelling to be freed. I was offered a sedative beforehand, but it came with a paper to sign that said one possible result of the drug was death, so I chose to pass it up. As it happened, I surprised myself: I didn't mind the MRI too much. My daughter was in the room with me, and the technician, Pedro, arranged a small mirror at the end of the long tube so that I could see her and not feel totally cut off from the world of the living. This was kind of him, but he couldn't get the mirror in exactly the right position, so I saw only a segment of her face, oddly angled, as in a Picasso painting.

After the MRI we had to wait a long time for an orderly to wheel me back to my room; it was the week of New Year's, so the hospital was understaffed. I was more than willing to walk but that wasn't permitted. I was starving and the candy machine in the hall didn't work. We asked Pedro if he had anything around to eat. He said apologetically that all he had were a few pretzels. He gave us an enormous plastic jar with a red top and a few pretzels way down at the bottom. We reached in, our arms in the jar practically up to our elbows. They were great pretzels—I can taste them to this day.

The preparation for the TEE is being done by a nurse with minimal English. One of the innumerable things I learned during my two five-day stays in different hospitals, one for the surgery and one for the TIA, is that the caretakers of hospital patients are nearly all immigrants. Why is this? Are immigrants particularly good at hospital care, or is it the only job they can get? We certainly should not complain about immigration because without it many of us might be dead or neglected. Not only nurses and attendants, but doctors as well (though not my all-American surgeon).

As with the angiogram, the preparation for the TEE takes a very long time, longer in fact than the test itself, and involves, among other things, the nurse spraying some foul-tasting stuff into my throat to numb it. She apologizes profusely for the taste, which I find puzzling: with a tube about to travel all the way down my esophagus to photograph the back of my heart, who gives a damn about a bad taste?

After a while the doctors arrive, a man and woman, both very young, the man wearing a yarmulke. They barely acknowledge me lying on their table, no more than one would greet a sausage (kosher, in his case) brought in on a plate for your breakfast, in fact maybe less, and they talk to each other in low tones. Maybe they're talking about me but then again they might equally be talking about football scores or last night's blind date or problems with their aging parents. The nurse continues to explain the procedure to me, so thoroughly that I could probably perform one myself in a pinch. Definitely a case of too much information, especially as there's a partial anesthetic so I won't be fully awake or aware in any case. They must be obeying a new law of full disclosure.

The key part of the explanation regards the tube. While the young doctors continue their murmuring, the nurse holds up her second finger and says, "We use a tube like this, about this size, to go down your esophagus with a little camera at the end." It is amazing where they can put cameras nowadays, but I reserve that line of thinking for later. I'm interested in this tube.

"You will swallow the tube," she says.

"You must be kidding." I don't actually say it, though.

Noting my consternation, the nurse says with a smile, "Are you good at swallowing big things, big pieces of steak or chunks of banana?"

"No!" It happens that I'm very bad at that sort of thing. Even large vitamins are uncomfortable to swallow. As the child of civilized parents, I was taught to chew. Moreover, ever since a teenager in our building almost choked to death on a melted cheese and sausage roll, I'm afraid of choking. Her father, seeing her turning blue, tried the Heimlich maneuver, and when that didn't work, he flipped her upside down and held her feet and shook her until the gob popped out of her throat.

But before I even deal with the prospect of swallowing a

tube the diameter of the nurse's finger, I am appalled that she addresses me in the future tense, employed as the imperative. The future tense in this context is worse than the imperative itself, which would be, at the proper moment, "Swallow the tube!" If she were very polite, she might add "please." "You will swallow the tube" is a prediction. How dare she predict what I can or will do? Well, I have to be culturally sensitive, even at this stressful moment; she's obviously not expert in the nuances of English tenses. Still, she could do better. There are plenty of preferable locutions she might have used. She might even have said, "Please try to swallow the tube. But if you can't, we can use an anesthetic to get it down."

She never mentioned that option, but I learned later from my brother, who had the same procedure, that with anesthesia they can get the tube down the throats of reluctant swallowers. I should have known. If they can take out your heart for a few hours then put it back in with a little piece of horse stitched on, getting a tube down your throat must be child's play. Anyhow, I have no memory of swallowing the tube. It must have gone down one way or another, though, because I remember very clearly its coming out. The sound. I felt and heard the tube emerge from the back of my throat with a soft pop, like a cork deftly extracted from a bottle of wine.

Besides the choking incident with the Heimlich maneuver and the upside-down caper, the other thing on my mind after the nurse said, "You will swallow the tube," was a terrific movie from Colombia I'd seen not too long ago, called *Maria Full of Grace*. A young girl, very beautiful, pregnant and in desperate need of money, agrees to work as a drug mule and fly to the United States with 62 pellets of cocaine in her stomach. Each pellet is 4.2 centimeters long and 1.4 centimeters wide. Naturally you can't just swallow them, one two three. You have to learn how, rehearse, and one of the most harrowing scenes in the movie is Maria being trained to swallow objects of that size. A man gives her enormous black olives to practice on, and at first she chokes and gags. But she's desperate, so eventually she learns to swallow the olives whole. Before her flight she swallows all 62 pellets. We see her do a few and infer the rest. Later she has to gather them when they come out the other end—this is not shown but left to the viewer's imagination. However distasteful, it can't be as bad as swallowing them, I suppose.

I thought of that poor girl swallowing all 62, while I had to swallow only one. Plus she was far from home and pregnant and moneyless. I should consider myself lucky.

Things turn out all right in the end for Maria, who delivers her cargo, has her baby and lives in an apartment in, I believe, Queens. Not so for a friend of hers on the same mission: one of the pellets bursts inside her and she dies an agonizing death.

The other movie that comes to mind, inevitably, is that old porn flick, *Deep Throat*, about a woman with astonishingly ample sexual capacities, but that was the last thing I wanted to dwell on at the moment.

All during the preparation the two murmuring doctors kept fussing over some equipment on a table. I wanted them to acknowledge my presence as something more sentient than a slab of meat waiting to be carved, so I said, "Do you actually do these procedures all day long?"

"Yes," the woman answered, barely looking up.

It was on the tip of my tongue to say something about the Nazi doctors; more than the tip, the words were nearly on my lips. After all, I thought, there's a certain superficial similarity: the Nazi doctors also performed sadistic procedures all day long, though without anesthesia. Of course, the crucial difference is that their goal was not to heal but to destroy. That difference is pretty crucial, no doubt about it. Enormously, infinitely crucial. But setting aside the goal, the activity itself seems not so different. I don't mean to compare myself to the victims, merely to note again the conundrum of similar actions with widely different motives—as in the contradictions of acting on the Hippocratic oath.

But then I noticed the yarmulke. That was what restrained me from commenting. I didn't want to offend this obviously Jewish doctor, an observant Jew. Strange as it seems, there I was, a slab of meat awaiting his instruments, at his mercy, and *I* didn't want to offend *him*. Not that I feared his retaliation—I gave him more credit than that. But because a remark like that would be in extremely poor taste, especially to a Jew. I was proud of my restraint. After the procedure was over, I told my husband and daughter, who were waiting outside, the little joke that I discreetly restrained, about the Nazi doctors. They were not amused. My husband said a remark like that would be in bad taste to any doctor, Jew or not didn't matter. I should keep such outrageous comparisons to myself. Had I not been lying exhausted on a gurney, he would have told me to develop some perspective, to see things in their proper proportions. He often tells me that when I'm in good health, and of course, he has a point.

All the medical people were pleased at the results of the procedure, which showed that I hadn't had a stroke; no little pieces of grunge matter had detached and swum to my brain. This was very good news to me too and I was happy, sort of. But my happiness was diluted by the imperative mood of the nurse's order—You will swallow the tube—which kept echoing in my ears. I suppose I'm oversensitive about language, and everything else.

For instance, I once tried to count how many people in

the hospitals had handled my body. How many hands? I felt almost like a prostitute, having been touched intimately by so many strangers—and not even getting paid for it. I got up to about fifteen, unsure whether I should count the aides who came in several times a day to take blood or take my blood pressure. Those aren't very intimate or intrusive procedures. But I decided to count them as well. Another uncertainty was how many people had been in the operating room during the surgery. I'd imagine three or four at the very least. If it took four to do the angiogram, probably there were more in the OR. "We reach in." Two to reach in and . . . and what? Remove the heart? Work on it in place? Another two to attach me to the heart-lung machine at just the right moment, before the brain is deprived of oxygen and lapses into vegetation. After a while I lost count, couldn't keep them all straight in my mind. Let's just say a lot of hands.

In between all these tests I would walk down the very long hall, south to north—it covered two city blocks—until I reached the big picture window at the north end. This second hospital was very near my home, only a block and a half away. I'd had dealings here before: I'd visited a neighbor with appendicitis and a friend's daughter who had a baby; I'd telephoned the public relations office to complain that employees arriving for the seven a.m. shift were shouting under my window, where they parked their cars. I'd been to the emergency room a few times, nothing serious, most recently for a mysterious black-and-blue blotch on my eyelid: the doctor suspected my husband had hit me but I assured him that wasn't so. I'd brought my children to the ER for the calamities of childhood—falling off a bike and losing a piece of a finger, getting a shard of glass in the foot . . .

So it was our familiar local hospital, and as I reached the north windows at the end of the corridor, I realized I could see my apartment very clearly, its southern side, living room, study, dining room and bedroom windows. I longed for wings, so that I could fly through the window and across to the comfort of my apartment. So near and so unattainable. "You are a patient."

By the end of the tests I found my thoughts turning to leeches. In many movies set in the nineteenth century, and in the many Victorian novels I read in college and afterward, there are scenes of sick people being treated with leeches that suck their blood. The patients lie on their stomachs and the leeches are applied to their backs. I was always sickened by the shiny black leeches, the bloodsuckers that would gorge themselves on bad blood. Watching them in films or picturing them while reading, I would begin to shift and shrug in my chair, feeling tiny tentacles scraping at my back. I felt so sorry for the patients treated in this way, and so superior too: look how ignorant people were then, they didn't have any better treatments, they didn't know the leeches were useless. (Although I believe I read somewhere recently that leeches do have some salutary effects.)

But after all the tests I had during my second hospital stay, I changed my mind. Enough of modern technology! Bring on the leeches!

Yeats and the Fear

Back at home, I gradually became aware of what I could and couldn't do. I grasped what I was now, I and my bit of horse. In a word, less: less in body and spirit—meaning muscle and mind—less in will and desire and capacity. How long this recovery would take, I had no idea, and I had no idea whether I would ever retrieve the "more" I'd once had, or been. Maybe like AA veterans, I would be "in recovery" for the rest of my life.

How changed I was: my constant thought. Some lines from the Yeats poem "Easter, 1916" kept going through my mind. "All changed, changed utterly. A terrible beauty is born."

Those lines were hyperbolically inappropriate for my situation: the poem is a memorial to the Irish rebels executed after their unsuccessful Easter uprising in 1916. Yeats names them at the end, a kind of incantation: "our part / to murmur name upon name / as a mother names her child / when sleep at last has come / on limbs that had run wild." It's a frustrated, brokenhearted poem, its rhymes and three-beat lines almost like a child's verse in contrast to its content. "All changed, changed utterly. . . ."

I first read Yeats when I was a graduate student. In a seminar on the great modern writers, we read Yeats for months, everything he ever wrote, including the automatic writing, which he said came to him from voices only he could hear. The teacher was dignified and ladylike in an old-fashioned way, with print dresses and white hair that looked like she'd just come from a beauty salon, and it was unsettling to hear her discuss the more ribald passages of Joyce's *Ulysses*. There were only three students in the seminar: besides me, an Indian woman who wore wonderful outfits, not saris, but trousers and long embroidered tunics in bright colors—I looked forward to seeing what she had on each Tuesday and Thursday; and a woman who was married with four children and lived right in the neighborhood. She became a close friend. She continued her studies and went on to teach at Bryn Mawr and eventually to become the head of the English Department, though she did not look or dress or comport herself in any way like our original teacher. It was in this friend's guest room that I discovered the mystery novels of Henning Mankell when I taught there years later.

Yes, I thought, changed utterly. Weaker, shakier, shrunken (I'd lost ten pounds, something I'd wanted to achieve for a long time, and now they were gone effortlessly), diminished in every way. But once again I was exaggerating mightily. What Yeats means by "changed" is not weaker or thinner but dead. "A terrible beauty" must refer to the beauty of the men's sacrifice for their ideals, for liberty, if one sees things that way. That sentiment is often invoked in wartime but I find it hard to accept. However, within the poem, I could accept it.

I was not dead for a noble cause. In fact, according to the cardiologist, I had been saved from possible death within the next couple of years. I tended to forget this, or maybe I'd never really believed it, since I hadn't had any pain or severe symptoms. I was, I am, insufficiently grateful. I'm well aware of that. On the contrary, I was willfully, ignorantly resentful. And there was nothing terribly beautiful about how I looked just now. Ten pounds less does not qualify as "a terrible beauty."

At one point I gave in to despair at my diminished self and moaned to a friend, "What did they do to me?" She was a tough sort who was discriminating with her sympathies. "What did they do to you?" she echoed curtly. "They saved your life. Have a little perspective." That again! I like those painters of the Middle Ages, before the Renaissance artists began rendering perspective from the human standpoint. Earlier, everything was flat and one-dimensional, in the same plane. I'm not ready to think in more planes than one, the most simplistic.

It occurred to me that just as future psychiatrists and psychotherapists must undergo analysis or therapy not only to know themselves, as Socrates advised, but to see how it feels from the patient's point of view, future heart surgeons, too, should undergo the procedures they will be performing. Maybe all of the resident surgeons in all of the disciplines, come to think of it: throat, lungs, liver, brain, intestines, whatever.

During my first couple of weeks at home I wasn't up to much activity, but I was determined not to sit idle. I deleted dozens of old emails from my computer, which I used in bed on a special board my daughters got me, which served as a desk. Deleting emails was so dull that I couldn't do it for more than twenty minutes at a time. I recopied our address book into a fresh, empty one. The entries of the people who'd moved many times, including one of our children, are now much neater, without all the crossing out and squeezing in of the new information. In the new book I omitted the people who had died. Most of them I'd already crossed out in the old book, but there were a few I hadn't had the heart to cross out, people I still felt close to: crossing out their names meant I accepted their deaths. Or was even indirectly complicit in them. I hadn't crossed out Rebecca or Glenda. But I omitted them from the new book. Writing them in felt too creepy: they were no longer at their old addresses or at any addresses I was aware of.

I was much visited. Visits from family and friends were pleasant, though they wore me out after about half an hour. I was visited a couple of times a week by a visiting nurse and by a physical therapist. The visiting nurse took my blood pressure, asked me questions and entered data in her computer. The physical therapist taught me exercises to get my muscles moving again. The exercises were absurdly simple, moving a leg or an arm a few inches in one direction or another. That I, with my years of modern dance, ballet and African dance classes, my daily half hour of stretches, my workouts at the gym on machines that resembled the torture instruments I'd seen in a museum of the Spanish Inquisition in Toledo (Spain, not Ohio)—that I should have to practice these infantile exercises (and find them difficult!) was mortifying.

When I told the cardiologist how tired I got when I did any exercise, he said I must push myself, to get back my stamina. Push yourself, he said firmly. If you get tired, sit down for a few minutes, have a glass of water, then get up and start again. Don't push yourself, said the physical therapist. Take it easy and never do too much. If you get tired or short of breath or your heart pounds, stop at once.

Some days I pushed and some days I didn't, but either way, those exercises and visits from the various professionals with their blood pressure kits signified that I was still a patient, even though I was in my own home and wearing my own clothes rather than the ugly white dotted gown. You are a patient, that nurse had said on the very first day. Her words had cast a spell, transformed me into a patient like a princess into a hag. What special charm could turn me back into an ordinary human being?

"Transformed utterly. A terrible beauty is born."

The poetry reflected my shock. This event had never been in my life plan; I'd been told my heart was strong. I was peripherally aware of aging, but I took for granted that my strength would carry me through indefinitely. Now that belief was destroyed.

If only a terrible beauty had been born from my surgery, but that was not to be. About two months after the operation, I was overtaken by waves of fear. Not quite tsunamis, but pretty big. They swept through my body; my heart with its new valve pounded; my joints and skin felt tense; my hands trembled so that my signature looked palsied, and I had the ominous sense that something bad was about to happen. These weren't ordinary anxiety attacks, which I'd never had, and which I've been told last a finite time, maybe twenty minutes. My spells were less intense, but could continue for an entire day. They were the inner ambience in which I spent my days.

I was back at work and trying as best as I could to resume the activities of my pre-surgical life. But now, with the fear, certain of those activities became impossible: I couldn't be with people, for one thing. The company of my fellow human beings took more composure than I could muster. Supermarkets were chaotic and bewildering. Subways were out of the question.

The anxiety that gripped and bewildered me, I learned, was a common repercussion of heart surgery. I never expected it. None of the doctors had mentioned it; it's hardly an inducement. Not that that matters much. I would still have had the surgery, and I doubt that anticipating massive anxiety would have made it any easier to bear.

Before, I'd occasionally felt what I casually called depressed, but I see now that that was a misnomer: I'd been merely unhappy or out of sorts or discontented, nothing that required medical attention. These new feelings were something else. Unimagined. As if I'd been colonized by aliens bringing unknown viruses and symptoms. In fact, the anesthetic I'd been under for five or six hours was an alien substance that would take quite some time to dissipate. Besides the anesthetic and the emotional trauma, there'd been that mysterious heart-lung machine that for several hours substituted for my real heart. No one seems to know exactly what effect that could have on post-surgical depression, or on anything else, for that matter.

I began each morning by looking forward to the evening, when the anxiety would ebb. Then I would carry my pillow and quilt to the living room couch and settle in with the three remotes to watch movies. I blessed Netflix. I read *War and Peace*. I wanted something that was sure to be good and would last very long. I'd read it when I was around nineteen or twenty but had forgotten most of it except that Natasha first loves Andrei and after he dies she loves Pierre. Surely there was more to it than that! *War and Peace* offered the uncanny comfort of rereading: some parts feel utterly unknown, and then as we go along, gradually a sense of familiarity begins to unfurl and blossom. We know and don't know at the same time. There's the thrill of stepping onto fresh territory, or rather territory we've visited before but which has renewed itself especially for our return visit.

I tried to explain to the doctors that I wasn't so much depressed as anxious. They said it was the same thing, anxiety, depression. I didn't see their logic but was in no condition to argue. ("Agitated depression," a doctor friend told me when I mentioned it. That little phrase made more sense.) I was again at the doctors' mercy: no longer a slab of meat in their hands but a vat of chemicals gone awry, to be treated with more chemicals, controlled substances that would counteract the uncontrolled chemicals within. They said it could last six months or more, but it would definitely go away someday. I couldn't imagine that. I couldn't remember how I used to be. Luckily I was able to walk to the drugstore to pick up the prescriptions, but waiting in line made me want to jump out of my skin.

I tried hard to think of what I was really afraid of. Everything, nothing. Everything unexpected that might happen in the next moment. Nothing I could name with certainty. I was afraid of fainting, of collapsing in the shower or walking down the street. I was afraid of facing my work. I was afraid of idleness. I was afraid when I was tired—and I was tired a lot of the time—but when I took naps, I was afraid I'd never manage to get up. (I did always get up.) I was afraid of life and afraid of death. But that's all there is—what other state could I retreat to?

When I pushed my questions further, I realized I was afraid of what had already been done to my body, even though that was over and I was no longer in pain. What exactly went on in the operating room while I was unconscious? That was the experience missing from my memory, making my mind unbalanced and plagued by uncertainty. I could easily have asked doctors or looked it up, but I preferred my lurid imaginings.

Lurid Imaginings

Forty or fifty years ago doctors didn't tell patients very much about their conditions, even when they were terminal. Doctors did not explain which procedures they resolved upon and why, or what symptoms or side effects might ensue. But over time patients began to assert their right to know, and so by now things have come full circle. They tell you everything. The scientific part, that is. My cardiologist, that kindly, balding, unflappable man, told me all about how aortic valves work, how mine was not working properly—he even pointed this out on a computer rendition of my heart in action—and how the new valve would perform better. I've forgotten the details, as I always forgot science lessons right after the exams, but for a while I understood how blood is pumped through the body, and why I was finding it harder to climb subway stairs and walk up hills. I had thought that was a symptom of aging and smoking, but no: it was my nasty valve reneging on its duty.

What intrigues me more than the biology, though, is how the surgery is carried out. The mechanical part. For instance, I have a pale pink line about seven inches long going down the center of my chest, starting about two inches below my collarbone: the scar. I don't mind the scar on aesthetic grounds and I'd never dream of trying to hide it: it's not especially ugly and hardly noticeable anyway. But when I see it in the mirror, I'm reminded that it was, for a few hours, a gateway of sorts. It is the mark of a double door opening to the secret lodging of my heart. "We reach in." Welcome to my inner life, I could have said, had I been conscious when the doors opened. Some double doors open automatically and majestically, but not these. How exactly did they open?

That's just one question I might have asked the surgeon when we met, had my mind not gone blank. Now I'm teeming with questions. How do you open someone's chest, that is, create the vertical slit that allows for the double doors? It must be with a plain old hammer and saw, right? The surgeon or one of his helpers must draw a line down the center of the chest, maybe with a pencil or a Bic pen, but they can't use the hammer right away. They must have to saw along the line first. Once they've sawed and sawed, scored the chest, as it were, then the surgeon can raise the hammer high and bring it down on the sternum like Paul Bunyan swinging his mighty axe. What does it sound like? Splitting wood? Or the kind of jagged, rough sounds you hear from the back of old-style butcher shops?

So the vertical line is broken, and maybe a few ribs and other parts too. The double doors are forced open to reveal the precious beating, pumping heart lying in its bloody chamber.

"We reach in."

Somehow they disable the heart and keep the body alive by means of the heart-lung machine. I wouldn't know how to begin asking about this machine. Is it attached to the heart? How? And also to the lungs? How big is it? Is the heart actually removed from the body? Does "reach in" mean reach in to extract the heart, or reach in to work on it? And if they do remove it, where do they put it for the hour, or two, or three that they're working? (I hope they're wearing gloves, by the way. Of course; nowadays even supermarket clerks wear gloves.) Is it on a table? In a special dish or bowl? How far is it from my body, where it usually resides? Does it feel anything—abandoned, say? What if someone is clumsy and the heart slips out of the bowl and slides along the floor? They run to rescue it. It sounds like a children's book: Catch Timmy's heart before it rolls down the hill. Is the little valve of horse sewn on with a needle and thread or attached some other way, staples, Velcro? How do they get the heart back in the chest in exactly the right position? Are the double doors of my chest open the whole time, the unaccustomed air wafting over my innards? Couldn't I catch a cold, so exposed?

I can't remember all of this, but I believe it happened, or something very like it. It still exists, on the dark side of memory. Memory has its dark side, unseen, like the dark side of the moon. Whatever is done to the body cannot be obliterated, only turned away and hidden.

Rehab

Among the mounds of printed material the hospital sent home with me was a progressive schedule of walking. You start out with two blocks a day and gradually increase until you're up to a mile a day. It was a very cold winter; I would bundle up to stroll along the park opposite our apartment. In the past I used to shiver in the cold, but no longer. It must have been the bit of horse, speeding my blood on its way faster than it had flowed in years. At first my husband or a friend walked with me, but soon I walked alone. I forced myself, even when the anxiety was enveloping and I feared I might collapse along the way and never make it home. In my worst fantasies, I was picked up from the snowy ground and sent back to the hospital to start all over again. When I arrived home safely from my walks, it was with great relief, as if I had survived a perilous journey, an expedition to the North Pole.

In the midst of my "agitated depression" I began an eight-week program of cardiac rehab three mornings a week at yet another hospital. There I found some half-dozen patients disporting themselves in a small gym in the basement, with the usual treadmills, stationary bikes and weight machines. The patients changed from week to week; some graduated, newcomers arrived. The women talked in the dressing room as women tend to do. (Maybe men do too, I don't know.) Undressing together seems to promote emotional and spiritual intimacy. One woman who looked older than I but was actually younger said she cried a lot of the time. A much younger woman said she was so wretched with her husband that she had to figure out a way to leave him. "Don't make major decisions when you're so depressed," the other woman and I both advised. Just as years ago, my friends and I would remind each other not to make any decisions when we had our periods.

The last step in the dressing room was to attach the intricate color-coded patches and wires to our chests so the nurse at a computer could keep track of our heart rates, and for all I know, our thoughts and feelings too. The program was me-

ticulously organized: each day we were given a personally tai-
lored schedule of which machines to use, for how long, and
at what rate of speed. The physical therapists were so kind
and efficient as to seem supernatural. One of them actually
resembled Wonder Woman.

Every so often a patient would report chest pains or diz-
ziness and would promptly be led to a wheelchair. Often that
patient was sent to the emergency room, and as he or she was
wheeled out, the rest of us, looking on, kept pacing on our
treadmills or hoisting our weights. This felt heartless, but
what could we do? It could be any of us in that wheelchair. It
was best to ignore it. Leave it to the professionals.

The program worked well: the more I exercised, the
stronger I got. It didn't help the fear, though. That would
take a long time to simmer down, if ever. (I can see in what
I've written here that some of the extreme feelings are a result of the fear. Though that doesn't mean I disown them.)
Beneath the fear was the sense of waiting, which outlasted
the fear. Waiting for something, though I never figured out
what. Maybe for the return of my former self. My former
strength, endurance, fortitude, courage.

As the weeks passed, I began to feel changes. This time I
wasn't changed utterly, only in small ways. I could walk up a
hill or up the subway steps without growing short of breath.
I could be with a friend for the duration of a brief walk. After
a while I could go to a restaurant or a movie without feeling
so restless that I had to flee. I became interested in the news
again, the wars and natural disasters. It was even conceivable
that, with patience, I would stop being a patient and repos-
sess the "more" I had once been. Yes, I might soon be restored
to life, a real life, and this real life would last longer than it
would have without the surgery. And as I tentatively began
to feel inhabited by this "real life"—going out to a movie,

talking to people in a café, caring about my work, enjoying family get-togethers—it was very like rereading *War and Peace* after a long hiatus: stepping into territory that was familiar and fresh at the same time, territory that was being renewed precisely by my own return.

It was still hard to admit that the surgery was a good thing. Now that it was over, I didn't want to think about it, good or bad. What I did think about was the horse, whom I imagined grazing in a green meadow under a blue sky. Before he gave up his heart valve, of course. It occurs to me: is it possible that horses are killed expressly for their valves, as in the illegal traffic in human organs? On that day when I first met the surgeon, did he call a stable and order a horse's valve? I wouldn't want to be the cause of any horse's death. Be that as it may, I am the beneficiary, and I feel grateful to the horse who pumps my blood so effectively.

I never smoked those two cigarettes I brought with me the first day. When I got home, I put the almost empty pack of Vantage in the bottom drawer of my night table, next to an unopened carton. They're still there, almost eight months later. Even though I probably won't smoke anymore (though you never know, I might regain my old nonchalance), I feel those two are owed to me.

My Mother Speaks

The Rubber Band Ball

When we were little, we made things from whatever came our way—we had no fancy toys like now—and one thing we loved to make was a rubber band ball. You know how rubber bands keep turning up, around asparagus or lettuce, brand-new pencils and envelopes, only to end up cluttering the kitchen drawer? Everything has a use. A rubber band ball is a wonderful thing.

First we'd ball up a bit of newspaper very tight, roll it around in our palms, get it nice and round, almost as big as a golf ball but not quite. The most important thing was very tight. We'd raid our mother's collection of rubber bands and wrap each one around the ball of paper, doubling or even tripling it, though it was best to start with a few small, fat and sturdy ones, and at first it looked like nothing, just a clump of paper with some rubber bands around it, then after a while— this needed time and patience—less and less paper was showing, till almost by magic—this was the best part—you'd see it becoming a real ball.

Once it took shape, it went so much faster and easier. You'd keep adding more and more, till all at once, the way it happens with a cake or soup, you knew it was done: There was a good firm ball you could bounce or throw. It bounced like a dream, as high as you ever could wish.

So I thought, here I am with time on my hands, I'll make

one for our girl, your little one. I started saving rubber bands and wrapping them around tinfoil—it holds together better. We didn't have it back then. I pictured her playing with the ball I'd made for her, bouncing it on the sidewalk like I used to do, but then I imagined what if she dropped it and it rolled into the street with all the traffic? She dashed after it just as a car was coming—my heart pounded so hard, I couldn't watch . . .

So I didn't make the rubber band ball after all. I couldn't, with what I had pictured in my mind. I had to throw it away. I was so relieved she wouldn't have it.

My Mother's Report When I Return from Work

So here you are. Everything's fine, she napped and woke up happy to see me. I gave her some spinach and a boiled egg, she didn't take much of her bottle but later in the park I got her a Dixie cup from the man in the truck and she liked that very much—she even tried to eat the wooden spoon. She only wanted to go on the slide with the big kids and cried when I wouldn't let her, but I pushed her in the baby swing and she liked that. You were short of milk, I saw, so we stopped for some.

The ironing's on the bed, I pushed the vacuum around, I hope you don't mind, the place looked like it could use it, and I did a load of diapers while she slept. You had a few calls, I wrote all the messages down, also a package came, looks like a book. After the park we played with her puzzle. Some smart kid, she knows where all the pieces go, she did it faster than I think I could. I gave her a bath, I knew you'd be tired after work—boy, can she splash around, I mopped the floor—she's in her pajamas now, all ready for bed. We read her book, she pointed at all the right pictures. Oh, and I roasted a chicken—for me that's no work—you'll have a head start with dinner so your husband won't have to wait.

I'll tell you something, I always thought a woman should stay home and take care of her baby. But in your case I see you can't. So all right, it was a very nice day and I'll see you next week. I suppose you'll manage till then?

The Renaissance

When I was thirteen, a year of such adolescent angst that I was sure it would be the worst year of my life, I started ninth grade. On the first day of history class, our teacher, Mr. Feigenbaum, told us about the Renaissance. Mr. Feigenbaum, whom I can still see standing beside his large wooden desk at the front of the classroom—I always had a seat up front because I was short—was also fairly short and wore a brown suit. He had dark hair thinning at the top, and glasses with thick dark rims. He wasn't heavy but pear-shaped. There was nothing remarkable about his appearance; he was the sort of person you might not notice on the street. But he became remarkable to me because he was the first person to utter the transformative word, Renaissance, in my presence.

He told us that in the fourteenth and fifteenth centuries in Europe, a dazzling phenomenon swept over the land, a re-awakening of love for art and beauty, above all the arts and legacy of the ancient worlds of Greece and Rome, along with a burgeoning of new art and thought. It was especially startling because, he told us, it came after a period of some centuries called the Dark Ages, in which all of Europe apparently slept. Under a spell, I thought. As in a fairy tale.

I pictured a dim world in which nothing ever happened, shadowy and crepuscular as if trapped in a prolonged, static twilight. Nobody did much of anything besides the daily chores necessary to stay alive, and these they did in the dark and in silence, riddled with ennui. Then all at once burst the dazzling dawn of the Renaissance. Brilliant golden light broke through the clouds, spreading over every obscure corner of Europe, and people woke from their torpor and the Dark Ages were over. Everyone started painting and writing and making sculptures. (I later learned that the Dark Ages were not as dark as I had envisioned: plenty went on, but for the purposes of ninth grade, the Dark Ages did not merit class time.)

I was tremendously excited by this news of the Renaissance, which I'd never had an inkling of. Besides being exciting in itself, the news gave me hope, since I was living through my own Dark Age, mired in boredom and fretfulness, feeling rejected and useless, quite without alluring prospects. I swore to remember for the rest of my life how miserable I'd been that year. Surely I could never feel such misery again.

And in fact I didn't. Naturally I've had far more serious troubles than those typical of adolescence. But I've never again had that unique thirteen-ish feeling. It's nihilistic. You don't know who you are or what you want to do with your life, and you can't bear anything or anyone in it.

It's common knowledge that adolescents become obnoxious, typically toward their parents, and the causes are common knowledge too, though I've always found some of them dubious. One of the ways of being obnoxious, perhaps more frequent in girls, is having contempt for one's mother. In reality, there was nothing contemptible about my mother. She was good-humored, forthright, and had a peaceable nature. She was sociable, indeed charismatic, and often had friends over to play a favorite game of that time, mah-jongg. It must have been all those admirable qualities that I scorned, because I was just the opposite. In my uncertainty about who I was and how I could tolerate living, I must have needed to cling tightly to my ill humor and secrecy and argumentativeness. I longed to flee, but where? How? I knew there was a world beyond my immediate and circumscribed surroundings, indeed right over the bridge in Manhattan, but I didn't know how to get to it. Or rather, I knew how, but was not yet permitted to make the subway trip on my own. If thirteen wasn't the worst year of my life, it was surely a dark age.

I found my mother's limitations intolerable and was often uncivil to her. My brother-in-law, who joined the family when I was ten by marrying my much older sister, and who was calm and even-tempered, a peacemaker like my mother, said to me, "Can't you at least be polite to her? She's your mother, after all. Can't you talk to her?"

"How can I talk to her?" I said. "She doesn't even know what the Renaissance is."

Now, it's true that subjects like the Renaissance were not discussed in my family. But in retrospect, it's likely that my mother had in fact heard of the Renaissance. She completed high school in Brooklyn and went on to secretarial school, though I doubt that the Renaissance appeared on the curriculum there. But they might have covered the Renaissance in her high school. Would it have been in the syllabus? Surely some teachers other than Mr. Feigenbaum knew about it. Even if my mother hadn't heard of it, she might have liked to; I could have told her. But that never occurred to me.

One reason this contempt for my mother feels odd today is that not so long before it began, or emerged—a mere few years—one of my favorite privileges was helping her prepare for her semi-weekly mah-jongg games when her turn came round to host them. I loved to set up the folding bridge table in the dining room and place the four chairs around it, while my mother busied herself in the kitchen putting candies and nuts in little bowls, a prelude to the coffee and cake that would be served when the game was over.

My mother's mah-jongg set was in a mahogany-colored box of a sort of alligator material, longer and narrower than an attaché case. It had two brass levers on the sides that you snapped to open it. Inside, the supplies for the game were neatly stacked in compartments, a niche for every item. I set out racks about twelve inches long for each player, on which they would line up their tiles. At one edge of each rack were four small brass posts, about two and a half inches high, for the hexagonal mah-jongg money, red, green, blue and yellow for different denominations, each about the size of a nickel, with a hexagonal hole in the middle. I slid the money onto the brass poles through the hexagonal holes. The poles had a joint about halfway up, so they could bend over at a right angle, to keep the money secure. These curious little joints charmed me; I jiggled them over and over, like bending an elbow.

Next I set a mah-jongg card at each of the four places. The cards, a little smaller than postcards, were folded, and opened into three sections with enigmatic lists on each of the six sides. The lists showed the combinations of tiles that made a winning hand. Although I became familiar with the game from watching, circling the table and peering over the women's shoulders, I never understood the hieroglyphics of the cards.

The tiles, a little larger than a pat of butter, were a buttery color, each with a design on one side: dot, crack, bam and wind. My favorite task was dumping them from the box onto the center of the table and hearing the delicate clinking sounds they made. Then I had to turn each one facedown, hiding their Chinese designs. This I loved to do. It was laborious, but I enjoyed watching my progress—order obliterating chaos. I've always liked repetitive, incremental tasks like that.

Before the women arrived, my mother would check my work to see that I'd done it all correctly, and I was always proud when I had. Then the doorbell began to ring: the players arrived, and after the greetings and some gossip, they would sit down, gather the facedown tiles and line them up on their racks.

And by some unbidden process, puberty, I suppose, and all that accompanies it, somehow this intimacy, this childhood delight in helping my mother, morphed into contempt at thirteen. One of the things I developed the greatest contempt for was the mah-jongg games. They struck me as the pinnacle of middle-class banality. One bam, three cracks, five dots, the women would call out all afternoon, then have coffee and cake and go home to fix dinner.

How pointless, compared to the Renaissance. Mah-jongg and the Renaissance came to represent for me polar modes of life, and I had no doubt which I was meant for, if only I could find it—as if it were tangible and resided in a place.

By the time I learned about the Renaissance, I had stopped helping my mother set up for the games. If I came home from school to discover an afternoon game in progress, scorn rose in my throat like bile. It was all I could do to greet the women cordially, as my very civilized mother had instructed me. I would have preferred to roll my eyes but didn't dare. I grabbed a handful of salted peanuts from one of the bowls and clattered upstairs to my room, where I flung myself on my bed and mused about the Renaissance.

It would come. It had to come. Once I was allowed to ride the subway alone, the spell would be broken. Like the youngest son in a fairy tale, I would set out to find my true destiny.

For My Father, Shaving

When my first book was published, I would imagine someone meandering through a bookstore and idly picking my book from a shelf or a table. Something about the title or the jacket pricks her curiosity, and then she (it's probably a she) looks at the author's name, doesn't recognize it but starts leafing through. After a couple of paragraphs she tucks it under her arm with an air of satisfaction and brings it to the counter. Watching this, I'm thrilled. I was writing for her all along.

But it may not happen this way anymore. It's a fantasy based on a vanished reality, like going out into the street and finding horse-drawn carriages. Nowadays I may be writing for someone clicking around on a computer and by some trail of links, like the red paint dabs on tree trunks along forest trails, she comes upon my book, and maybe decides to take a chance and with a click, she tosses my book in. But that's unlikely, with all the choices at her disposal.

No, anything I write now will have to be for my father, standing at the bathroom sink, shaving. That morning of his shaving is not a fantasy, but it can never happen again. Some people are spurred on by recognition and praise and I am, alas, one of them. Or, more accurately, everyone is spurred on by praise and recognition, but some can continue well enough without it. I envy and esteem them but will never be one of them, and it is too late to try to fortify my character toward that goal.

I was seven years old, an early-morning moment, standing at the bathroom door, holding a sheet of lined notebook paper, torn out so that its side edges were jagged, bits of the torn edges fluttering in the steamy air from the bathroom. I had just finished one of my first stories and rushed down the hall with the page in my hand. This I brought to my father while he was standing at the bathroom sink, the door open as usual for his shaving ritual, a white towel wrapped around his middle like a mini skirt, the knot at the waist tucked in, the bottom half of his face covered in white lather, the razor in his hand. I must have been quite excited with what I'd done, if it couldn't wait until he had dressed and come down for breakfast.

But why him? The whole scene, the sheer presumption of the child, suggests a father far more patient and forbearing than I remember mine to be. I mostly remember him shouting and slamming doors. Somehow he was also the kind of father I felt free to interrupt in this manner.

Why didn't I bring the sheet of paper to my mother? She was probably up, dressed, and already preparing breakfast downstairs. She might have said, In a few minutes, sweetheart, let me get breakfast on the table. My older sister? No, she wouldn't have done at all; she would have been kindly but patronizing, and obviously absorbed by her own affairs, starting college, with her gorgeous smooth hair in a pompadour and her boyfriends with cars. My brother could not read. Indeed, he would not be born for several months. Even so, my father seems an odd choice. He spoke with eloquence and brio but wasn't particularly literary, though he read a great deal, books on politics and economics, not that his reading choices would have meant anything to me one way or the other. My mother was the one who read stories, love, romance, popular family sagas that she got from the lending library a few blocks away for two cents a day, with me accompanying her, holding her hand. Still, my father was the one I instinctively sought out, to show what I had done. Maybe because one of his favorite expressions was, There's no substitute for brains, a slogan I later came to despise and still do. There are many qualities more important than brains; even back then I suspected that. But I knew that in his eyes my story would show brains. Later I learned that brains are not what make a writer. Imagination does that, and need and perseverance and some luck thrown in.

There I stood at the bathroom door in my pajamas—it must have been a Sunday, yes, because I was in no hurry to get ready for school. Had it been a school day I would not have been writing so early, would rather have been anxious about getting ready in time to meet my friends outside and walk the six blocks, which this year, second grade, our mothers allowed us to do on our own; there were no broad streets to cross; anxious about lining up in the schoolyard waiting for the bell; anxious because of the nausea brought on by my intense dislike of school. Second grade was better than first, because despite having to line up in front of the classroom for Miss Shapiro to inspect us—teeth, fingernails, ears, hair, neck (we'd pull our shirts and dresses away from our necks to reveal the collarbone), and presence of a handkerchief (in the case of girls folded into a triangle and pinned to the chest of our dresses—how could we ever use it?), we no longer, as in first grade, had to go around the room and recite what we had for breakfast, which for me was a spur to creativity: I began my school career by throwing up my breakfast daily, so my mother had stopped urging food on me. Instead I would invent what I considered healthy and well-rounded breakfasts based on the posters hung around the room, always slightly afraid my lies would be found out. It never occurred to me to tell the truth and say, Nothing, for then we would all have gotten a lecture about the importance of breakfast and the seven food groups, than which few things were duller.

So it wasn't that kind of day, it was a blessed weekend day, and my father could take his time shaving, no need to put on his suit and tie and shiny shoes, eat a piece of toast and drink a cup of coffee standing up in the kitchen, holding his briefcase, then kiss everyone good-bye and rush off, and in a moment we would hear the familiar energetic rumble of the car, hear it roll out of the driveway and turn, often with a slight screech, into the street and off, away into the world. Because he wasn't in a rush, my father could turn away from the mirror and gaze down on me, listen to my request that he read my offering, at which point he put the razor down on the edge of the sink, dried his hands on a towel, not the one wrapped around his middle but one hanging from a rack, take the sheet of paper and read it. I could see he was really reading and not pretending—his eyes were moving from left to right and looked focused. I couldn't gauge the expression on his face because most of it was white with lather.

After a while he handed it back to me and I could see he was smiling amid the lather. "This is good," he said. "Very, very good."

The memory ends there, at its climax. I probably returned to my room and hid the paper somewhere, put on my clothes and carried on with the day. But the day could not get much better. Indeed the critical reception of my work could not get, and has not gotten, much better than that.

However pleased he may have been with my early display of talent, he did not hesitate, several years later, to put me in an uncomfortable position because of it. I showed him another story I wrote—not at the bathroom door but in the living room after dinner—a story that was a homework assignment. I recall only that it involved suspense: would someone get somewhere in time, catch an essential train. . . . It was the evening before I was to hand it in, and I needed not only his unfailing praise, but a title, which eluded me. He read the story and seemed absorbed by it. Why don't you call it *Tempus Fugit*? he suggested. Strangely, I didn't ask what this meant; I just asked how to spell it and wrote it at the top of the page. He seemed quite amused by the whole business, not only my story but the title he'd come up with.

The next day in school I was asked to read the story aloud, and after I had done so, the teacher asked me what the title meant. I had no idea. I was mortified. Why hadn't I thought to ask? I'm not sure the teacher knew either. If she did, she didn't say. Later, at home, I asked my father, and he told me: Time Flies. I had a heavy feeling in my chest, but not until much later did it occur to me to be angry at his little joke at my expense. I understood that, like me, he liked to show off. Yet why would he play this trick? And besides that, how and when did he learn Latin in the first place? He came to this country at the age of twelve knowing Russian and Yiddish and now spoke English perfectly and elegant-ly, accent-free, which must have taken some time. Latin too? Where did that fit in?

So, I finally grasped, this streak of nastiness could come from the same person who had praised my early story. It came from the same person whose frequent temper tantrums made the living room chandelier shake, who would dash out the door shouting at my mother, "You make my life misera-ble!" and drive away—the familiar rumble of the engine but angrier, the roll out of the driveway screechier—leaving me to wonder whether he meant miserable just for the moment when he uttered the words or miserable all of the time?

Lying on my bed with the door closed, I pondered which

of them I would choose to live with if and when they got divorced. I imagined that was imminent. I weighed the pros and cons. It was a close call. One thing was certain: my father would take me to restaurants more often and we'd eat the forbidden foods, like shrimp and pork chops and fried clams. But could that make up for the ugly words in his snarling voice?

My pondering was unnecessary: he always returned. Was it because the fit had passed, or because divorce was unheard of in our milieu? In any case, the choice was hard. Both my parents understood who I was when I was nine or ten, and both were indulgent and generous. But he knew me as a writer. I usually planned to go with him.

Degrees of Separation

Back in the 1940s, my family moved into a brand-new house in the Flatbush section of Brooklyn, neither then nor now one of Brooklyn's chic neighborhoods. It was a two-story attached brick row house identical to its neighbors. Modest, middle-class, affordable, a compact congenial house with a small front and back porch, front steps bordered by a tiny strip of grass, a driveway with a wall that would prove useful for handball. My father was proud that he could make the move and announced to everyone he knew that he was living in a Trump home.

I remember moving day quite well. The house had casement windows in the living room that opened on to the front porch, and our piano, dear to my mother and later to me, was maneuvered in through those obliging casement windows. Three small girls around my age—today they wouldn't be allowed out without a parent—stood on the sidewalk watching the piano caper and immediately offered to be my friends. That and the casement windows in every room and the three chimes in the living room that trembled when someone rang the doorbell endeared the house to me. I grew up there, and whenever my father made his announcement about living in a Trump home, I imagined Mr. Trump as a bountiful kindly gentleman, rather like Mr. Carmichael in *A Little Princess*, who supplied deserving families with nice places to live.

Only when Fred Trump's son Donald became a presidential candidate, arriving like a plague of locusts, except that locusts are expected periodically and Donald was not—did I start to wonder who exactly this Fred Trump, our longtime landlord, was? What did Donald come from?

Fred Trump, the son of German immigrant parents, started out in real estate at the age of fifteen. Too young to sign checks, he needed his mother to do it for him. He became one of the largest developers in Brooklyn, comparable in scale to the better-known Sam LeFrak in Queens. Donald liked this arrangement: "This way, I got Manhattan all to myself!"

During and after World War II, Fred Trump claimed to be of Swedish descent; as one of his associates put it, many of his tenants were Jewish and it wasn't a good idea just then to be German. Trump *père* died in 1999 at the age of ninety-three with an alleged fortune of $250 to $300 million. His lengthy *New York Times* obituary called him "one of the last of New York City's major postwar builders" and also remarked on his "silent-movie star" looks (not inherited by his son). In addition to Flatbush, he owned houses and apartments all over Brooklyn: Coney Island, Bensonhurst, Sheepshead Bay, Brighton Beach, as well as some in Queens, many of them intended for returning veterans.

In 1954 (while I was still living in the house), Fred Trump was investigated by a Senate committee for "windfall profits" made by acquiring ill-gotten loans from the Federal Housing Authority. This news was dismaying; it destroyed my fantasy of the small-time benevolent builder, and my family as the lucky recipient of his largesse. (Asking around now, I find that many people knew the scope of Trump's empire, while I had kept my childhood illusions.) Plus I didn't relish feeling any connection, however remote, to Donald Trump.

In 1973, the Justice Department's Civil Rights Division sued Fred Trump for discriminatory rental practices; his employees were instructed not to rent to black families and to keep applications coded by race. These practices were unearthed by the Urban League's fair housing program, which sent white testers to apartments denied to black applicants. When the white tester was offered the apartment, the agent was caught red-handed, as it were.

This fact alone wouldn't have surprised me, given the rental policies of those times. What was surprising was yet another degree of proximity. For in the late 1960s, I worked at that very same fair housing program, run by the indomitable Betty Hoeber, who nearly single-handedly forced landlords large and small to obey the laws, and cleared the way to a more integrated city. I worked as a checker, and I advised black families on where to look for housing. I followed cases we brought to the City's Commission on Human Rights. Had I not left to return to graduate school in 1970, I might very well have gotten involved in the case against the elder Trump, which resulted in his being forced to advertise apartments in minority newspapers and to list them with the Urban League.

All of this cast a cloud over the memory of the unprepossessing but comfortable house I grew up in. Nowadays I feel a bit of a shudder when I recollect my father's assertive voice boasting that he lived in a Trump home. We enriched the Trump family fortune for nineteen years.

What I Don't Know

When in my reading I come across sentences like this one, "Her great-great-grandfather was the principal advisor to the Dutch royal family in the 18th century; a great-grandfather made a killing in the gold rush, and her mother was descended from George Sand," I feel a trifle bereft. I don't crave the descendants' social position or wealth, simply their extensive location in history, going back centuries that for me are blank, as if my family sprang from nowhere. Of course my forebears must have existed in those centuries, but who were they, and what and where? Nobody tells.

There is no shortage of information about my twelve pairs of aunts and uncles, transplanted from Eastern Europe, and my twenty-six first cousins, born here and mostly gone now. Rumor, usually in the voice of my mother, had it that one uncle killed a pedestrian while driving; another, a doctor, gave his wife a lethal abortion. A cousin left her husband of one day for another man; another was shot to death by his Cuban refugee wife. One headed west to escape his humble origins, and one because he was secretly gay. And so on. Some of the stories are tragic, some the ordinary sprinkling of drama in any large family, from anywhere. They have the piquancy of gossip, yet they do not intrigue me. What I wonder about is the unknown earlier world, the past in which suffering was a daily event on a mass scale. So awesome that it mustn't be spoken of. Like the name of God, which religious Jews never write in its entirety, only abbreviated.

In a talk to a group of students, Grace Paley said, People always tell you to write what you know. No, she said, you should write what you don't know about what you know. For me that is a wide barren stretch, blank pages.

What I know for sure is that my ancestors did not come over on the *Mayflower*. My grasp of family history goes back only to my grandparents on either side, with the name of an occasional great-aunt or -uncle thrown in. For instance, I was told of an uncle of my father's named Peter, who went from his native Ukraine to Jerusalem (how, when?), where he worked as an architect. So on a trip to Israel I looked him up in histories of local architecture but with no luck. I thought he might have been part of the Bauhaus group that flourished in Tel Aviv in the 1930s, and I visited a neighborhood known for its many examples of their work. I strolled down the boulevard lined with handsome Bauhaus buildings, but nothing suggested my great-uncle or brought me closer to him. Maybe it was all a story.

Then for a while there was a family suspicion that we were related to Ariel Sharon, former Israeli general and prime minister. Sharon was my father's family's last name, shortened at Ellis Island from an unwieldy Yiddish name, as Ariel must have changed his, though not at Ellis Island. My mother insisted that Ariel resembled my father's brother George (a fat George, she called him), which notion his photographs supported, and his aggressive temperament fit well with my father's family. But a bit of research showed there was no connection. I'd had vague fantasies about introducing myself and through him meeting important Israelis. But in the end I was relieved; the possibility made me uneasy.

My father's parents came to the US early in the twentieth century on a ship whose name I don't know, nor do I know from which port in Europe it came. Has anyone ever investigated those ships that brought immigrants from Ireland and Italy and Eastern Europe? What were their names—the names of ships are always colorful. How seaworthy were they, I wonder. Did any sink, with their hopeful boatloads?

I don't know how my father's family got from Kyiv, their nearest city, to that European port. I don't know if they all came at once or in groups of two or three—there were the parents and eight children. The oldest son remained near Kyiv: I heard a vague story that he was already married with a family and was established in some career related to music; I like to imagine he was a pianist because I play the piano, but I really don't know.

I asked my mother if this oldest brother had kept in touch; she said for a while he sent letters and then they stopped coming. Did my father miss him? I couldn't imagine asking my father about him. He never spoke of his first eleven years. It was as if they had never happened, which was perhaps what he wanted to believe. Indeed it is hard to imagine my father, with his elegant, perfect English, in his neat suit and tie ready for work, or behind the wheel of his DeSoto, in some dusty shtetl maybe with chickens hopping around.

At twenty-one I was planning my first trip to Europe. I asked my father, who seemed profoundly uninterested in my plans, "Don't you ever want to travel? Like, don't you ever want to go to Europe?" "I've been to Europe," he said, in a way that promptly shut me up. He was bitter. To send his five sons to a good school in Kyiv, my Jewish grandfather had to pay four times the ordinary tuition for each, my mother told me. And, she said, the boys had to wear a yellow star, which shocked me because I thought that began with Hitler, decades later. But in fact the "badge," as it was called, originated in the Middle Ages, in various shapes and colors.

Irrelevantly, she added that my father would never eat

a banana because it was not something he knew from his youth. This was curious because in all the years since my father emigrated as a boy of eleven, he surely ate many things he had never encountered in childhood, such as fried clams and lobsters, which he and I would eat at Coney Island while my mother, who kept our home kosher, fled to the mountains for the summer.

For a long time, after I learned about the war and the concentration camps (from books, not from my parents), I assumed the Nazis must have thrown this oldest brother and his family into the ditch at Babi Yar among 33,000 others, an incident made famous by the Russian poet Yevgeny Yevtushenko in his 1961 poem protesting the Russian government's refusal to acknowledge the deed. But shortly before she died, my older sister, an occasional source of information, said she'd heard this brother and his family might have emigrated to Israel.

Which was it, Babi Yar or Israel?

Some years ago one of my father's brothers made a family tree to give to the younger generation. From this tree I learned that my paternal grandfather, whom I had known as a small wizened old man shuffling around a three-room apartment in Brooklyn, who spoke no English but could read it, had once been a steward for the estate of a Polish nobleman. I don't know if this was an important position or nothing much; whatever I know about stewards is from old novels or Chekhov stories. I suppose it depends on the size of the estate. Did he supervise serfs, I wonder, like the serfs in Tolstoi's stories?

From the family tree I learned that the maiden name of my father's mother, a small wrinkled gray-haired woman who smelled of rotting apples—not bad, a kind of sweetish smell—was Nuzzi, an Italian name. Since I have always wanted to be Italian, I seized on this information with enthusiasm. Someone told me it was a north Italian name. I checked with Ancestry.com—only the chance of my having Italian genes would make me spit into a tube and mail it—but it turned out there was nothing Italian in my DNA, only Eastern European and a couple of remote percentages so small I've forgotten them. I sometimes invent stories about how my grandmother came by that name.

I don't remember her death, but I recall vividly learning of my grandfather's death. I was six and walked the five short blocks home from school with friends. I opened the front door, and instead of finding my mother, I found my seventeen-year-old sister, all dressed up, her hair in a pompadour, sitting in a large throne-like chair with elaborate wood carving, a chair that faced me as I walked through the living room. She was sitting very still and somber. She had a flair for the dramatic. "Zadie died," she announced grimly, and it was clear to me even then how much she was enjoying the drama of the moment and the role assigned to her, to be home when I returned from school and convey the news. It didn't mean much to me—I knew Zadie as the severe old man who, according to my mother, had been a harsh disciplinarian and learned to read English by studying the *New York Times*. All I recall about his death is the image of my sister, stately, dressed suitably funereally, occupying the big chair as though she were royalty.

I know even less about my mother's parents, not even where in Eastern Europe they came from. I'm not sure my mother herself knew—she was one of the younger children born here; for her, life began in calm Williamsburg in Brooklyn. Without any bitter history to bury or repress, she was not as chary with information as my father. She said her father crossed the ocean on his own and established himself in

Manhattan with a pushcart, selling old clothes, before sending for his wife and two daughters. While she waited to be summoned, my grandmother, a charismatic and enterprising woman, the sort people call a force of nature, ran a hardware store back wherever they came from. I would have liked to ask her about running the store, but though we communicated in some fashion using Yiddish and English, neither of us was fluent enough in the other language to discuss the intricacies of the hardware business.

At the time I was born, my maternal grandparents lived in a five-story brownstone in Brooklyn, with each of their four daughters and their families occupying a floor. How this family and all the others like them managed the travel arrangements, the slow air mail letters, the packing, procuring tickets, trekking to a seaport, is a mystery. Another mystery is how my grandfather progressed beyond a rickety pushcart to owning that sturdy brownstone.

But the mystery that nags most is about my unknown uncle: Babi Yar or Israel?

The Other Henry James

In 1913, three years before his death, Henry James sat for a startling series of photographs. Probably because they were studies for a bust to be made by a young sculptor, they show no attempt at the usual dignity. James wears a limp, collarless shirt and vest; his huge dome of a head looks ready to burst with what he knows; his features are thick with resignation, his eyes pouched and darkly meditative; the broad cheeks sag, the neck is grooved. He seems not exactly defeated but nakedly worn out by his labors, a man who's spent the best of himself and is no longer certain why. The photos are as different from the familiar magisterial ones as *The Other House* is unlike his familiar great novels.

Why have we never heard of *The Other House*? At least I had never heard of it even though, in my English major and graduate school days, I put in time and a half at the James shrine. Nor had all but one of the half-dozen literate friends I polled. Was it some indiscretion critics had conspired to hush up? Had it thudded into obscurity by its own weight, or drifted off by its weightlessness?

The germ of the story came to James in December 1893, in the midst of his ill-starred playwriting phase. Typically, he seizes on it and starts shaping it in the *Notebooks*: a vow of fidelity made to a dying wife; a Good Heroine and Bad Heroine both in love with the widowed hero who's sworn not to remarry (how James loves, in one way or another, to bar his characters from marrying); a poisoned child. Somehow all ends well: the "poison," by a plot maneuver, turns out to be harmless; the child wakes up.

James was enthusiastic about his melodramatic nugget: "the 1st chapter of my story—by which I mean the 1st act of my play!" There's the operative word—"play." He sketched out a three-act scenario called *The Promise*, with the female lead probably intended for Elizabeth Robins, who had been playing Ibsen heroines on the London stage during the early 1890s. Like many of his contemporaries, James was much taken with Ibsen. Indeed, Leon Edel and other critics suggest that he conceived his passionate and complex bad heroine, Rose Armiger, as a kind of Hedda Gabler. When James abandoned the theater in horror after the shocking reception of his play, *Guy Domville*, *The Promise* was put aside.

Genius can be perverse. Why else would James have stubbornly craved success as a playwright, when the stage was about as uncongenial a place for his ruminating talents as a football field or a gambling casino? From 1890, with over a score of tales and a dozen novels to his name, among them *The Portrait of a Lady*, *The Bostonians*, and *Washington Square*, he devoted five years to writing plays. Two were produced. The first, an adaptation of his 1877 novel, *The American*, ran for a fairly respectable seventy performances. The second, *Guy Domville*, an eighteenth-century "costume play," precipitated what James would call "the most horrible hours of my life."

More than a century later, the famous fiasco loses none of its awfulness. James spent opening night, January 5th, 1895, seeing Oscar Wilde's *An Ideal Husband* and repaired to the St. James Theatre in time for the closing curtain of his own play, unaware of the jeers that had interrupted the hero's speeches. The producer and star, George Alexander, for reasons of his own, led James onstage, where he endured fifteen minutes of hoots and catcalls mingled with some valiant but unavailing applause. Imagine that hypersensitive, supremely worldly yet in some ways clueless soul facing such an uproar: it must have been like the massacre of innocents. And why did he stand there so long, anyway? Some rarefied notion of honor?

Less well known is that the eruption was later rumored to be the work of a claque with some grudge against Alexander. And that *Guy Domville* was politely if not lavishly praised by a number of critics, including George Bernard Shaw, and ran calmly for four more weeks. No matter, the damage was done.

James was crushed and renounced the theater for the time being. He pulled himself together, though: "I take up my old pen again—the pen of all my old unforgettable efforts and sacred struggles. To myself—today—I need say no more. It is now indeed that I may do the work of my life. And I will." And he did: over the next eight years he wrote seven novels, beginning with *The Spoils of Poynton* and ending with the great triad of *The Ambassadors*, *The Wings of the Dove*, and *The Golden Bowl*.

But before that efflorescence came *The Other House*. It might not have existed but for an 1896 invitation by the editor of the *Illustrated London News* to contribute a "love-story." The temptation is easy to see: fresh from his humiliation, James wanted to feel wanted; he wanted money, he wanted the wide audience that read the illustrated papers. How about that old scenario? Why not fix it up and get it into print, never mind how or where? He dug out *The Promise* and began reworking it for serialization. But he found, to his grief, that a play can't be transformed into a novel simply by rewriting the stage directions as narrative. "In an evil hour," he wrote to Edmund Gosse:

> I began to pay the penalty of having arranged to let a current serial begin when I was too little ahead of it, and when it proved a much slower and more difficult job than I expected. The printers and illustrators overtook and denounced me, the fear of breaking down paralyzed me, the combination of rheumatism and fatigue rendered my hand and arm a torture . . .

But he came through, despite conflicts with the editor over the illustrations, which must have appalled him: the handsome hero with dark mustache; the bad heroine holding a cup of poison—even after James changed her poison to drowning; a shadowy Satan lurking behind her, whispering in her ear. *The Other House*, as it was now called, was finished in haste, with the British and American editions coming out the same year.

Two contrasting houses are emblematic of rigor and laxity. One is stately, reliable Eastmead, presided over by Mrs. Beever, a banker's widow who, like her furniture, is "so 'early Victorian' as to be prehistoric." The mother of slow, ungainly, but good-hearted Paul, she has his future bride, the Good Heroine Jean Martle, all picked out. In the neighboring but very other house, Bounds (where the people are out of bounds), lives Tony Bream, a type James portrays with canny panache: while far from nouveau riche—Tony is Mrs. Beever's friend and partner in the old, rock-solid bank—his furnishings are suspiciously new and fashionable; his nature is a touch too readily accommodating, his manners too smooth. Tony is honorable, but his constant charm makes him dangerous: women fall in love with him; he likes it and lets them. In James's world, this amounts to irresponsibility, with fatal results.

For the most significant change from his original idea

is that the child victim does in fact die—offstage, which is just as well. Murders of the spirit and psychological terrorism abound in James, but a crime complete with corpse and villain makes *The Other House* unique. Leon Edel takes the "murder of innocence" to be purgative, "as if some remote little being within James himself had been 'exterminated' by the audience during that crucial night a year and a half earlier." If so, James might have attempted to give the child some reality: more prop than character, the prettified, mute four-year-old passed from lap to lap is hardly a satisfying vehicle for catharsis.

The crime is committed out of rampant passion: a woman wants a man so badly that she'll remove the impediment with her bare hands, hold the body underwater until it goes limp. This is far beyond what Kate Croy would be willing to do to Milly Theale in *The Wings of the Dove*—though as it happens, Rose Armiger, James's most wicked female conniver, is a precursor of the more circumspect Kate; for a really great novel, she had to be tempered and refined, like sugar.

True to its roots, *The Other House* reads like a play fleshed out with detailed stage directions: "Gradually, as she talked, he faced round again; she stood there supported by the high back of a chair, either side of which she held tight." Books First, Second, and Third correspond to three acts, set in a drawing room, a garden, and another drawing room, with characters coming and going, mostly in twos and threes, twining and untwining their intricate relationships. The scenes, or chapters, are crowded with incident and end abruptly at cliff-hanging moments, usually when a new character enters, as in French drama.

Book One, set in Bounds, opens with a shameless pretext to set the plot in motion. Tony Bream's wife, dying offstage after childbirth, insists that he vow not to remarry. Grief-stricken, he agrees, knowing her demand comes less from jealousy than from her miserable childhood at the hands of a stepmother. At the urging of the wife's old friend, Rose Armiger, the promise is morbidly modified to last only for the lifetime of the newborn child. Enter Rose's fiancé, Dennis Vidal, fresh from two years in China, with excellent financial prospects. But Rose, wagering on the wife's death and her own chances with Tony, sends Dennis packing.

Book Two, set in Mrs. Beever's garden four years later, offers one of the most delectable tangles James ever concocted. Young Paul Beever loves Rose (who loves Tony) but is under mother's orders to propose to Jean, who turns him down because she, too, loves Tony. Tony returns Jean's love but can't marry anyone, which hasn't prevented him from occasionally seeing Rose in London, maybe even sleeping with her— with James, one never knows. To complicate matters, Rose's jilted suitor returns. In a cold, controlled panic, Rose drowns young Effie and tries to frame Jean for the crime, leaving the way clear for herself and Tony.

A lot of plot—and that's the simplified version.

The denouement, in swift, fraught scenes, is a shocker. Soon enough, everyone figures out who the culprit is; with the help of the family doctor, they conspire to have Rose whisked away by Dennis. The crime goes unpunished. "Her doom," Tony tells the outraged Jean, "will be to live." Leon Edel was outraged too, and charged that the ending "defies the tradition of murder stories."

Rose doesn't regret her crime; like James, she doesn't seem to grasp it as a physical fact. She regrets only having failed of her purpose. For in time, we're given to understand, Tony and Jean will marry: the rather heavy irony is that Rose has successfully removed the child who was their obstacle.

James had high hopes. He wrote his brother, William,

that the novel showed "symptoms of being the most successful thing I have put forth for a long time. If that's what the
idiots want, I can give them their bellyful." He was mistak-
en. While the novel did go into a second edition, it wasn't
reprinted until 1947. Most later critics treated it with perfunctory dismissals: it gets three passing mentions in F. W.
Dupee's 1951 biography and two lines in Fred Kaplan's 1992
study, *The Imagination of Genius*.

Those who did comment found it "distinctly unpleasant,"
"inhuman," even "the one altogether evil book that he ever
wrote." (Were the others only partially so?) Edmund Wilson
was succinct: "Dreadful." A few critics, following Edel, saw it
as the projection of James's own trauma, a kind of Slough of
Despond on his artistic pilgrimage: "Without such a sojourn
in the abyss as it represents he would never have attained to
the full-bodied affirmation of the last and greatest period."
Thus the born-again theory of literary evolution.

And then *The Other House* returned from the abyss in a
new *New York Review Books* edition. Should anyone bother
to reprint it? To read it?

Yes, and definitely yes. Not for the anomaly of the murder, which plenty of lesser writers do far better. But for the
devilishly tortuous situation, first of all. (Who would have
thought we'd read James for plot?) For the ferocity of the
heroine's passion. Above all for the instructive spectacle of
genius on a bad day.

Precisely because it is misguided and abstracted in parts,
this peculiar novel about the potency of evil serves up James
raw rather than cooked, so to speak. Just as the late photos
reveal what youth and pride might have taken pains to conceal, *The Other House* shows his falterings and blind spots
alongside his subtlety and convolution: for one thing, heady,
analytic dialogues while a small soggy corpse lies in the next

room are preposterous. More happily, it demonstrates what he could do so innately well that no bitterness or haste or desperate ambition could impede it. Genius may be perverse, but it's also irrepressible.

The Other House contains some of the most harrowing, compressed, and ambiguous scenes James ever wrote. Take Rose's tense predicament when Dennis first returns to claim her: she must delay her answer while she waits to learn whether Tony's wife will die in the next room—that is, whether a better opportunity is about to open. She holds off the entreating Dennis with seductive agonies of teasing until he cries out:

"You're not sincere—you're not straight ... You're only gaining time, and you've only been doing so from the first. I don't know what it's for—you're beyond me; but if it's to back out I'll be hanged if I'll give you a moment."

In the face of Rose's obfuscations, this straight talk is enormously effective. What Dennis can't know, but a clever reader of thrillers might, is that Rose already has a glimmer of the crime she'll commit four years later, in hopes of winning Tony.

Their scene together after the murder is an even better mix of maddening duplicity and startling frankness, as sly Rose manipulates Dennis into shielding her with an alibi. James leaps from his wildly hermetic mode—

"'You like it [his loyalty, I think] so much on your side that you appear to have engaged in measures to create it even before the argument for it had acquired the force that you give such a fine account of'"—to exchanges like:

"If I count on you, it's to support me. If I say things, it's for you to say them."

"Even when they're black lies?" Dennis brought out. Her answer was immediate.

"What need should I have of you if they were white ones?"

The juxtaposition makes for fireworks—a bit showy, sure, but irresistible.

The climactic confrontation between Rose and Jean is a barely veiled catfight, while Effie, with only minutes left to live, sits placidly imprisoned on Rose's lap. Plotting to deflect suspicion, Rose confounds her rival with lies and insinuations that Jean herself might kill the child out of passion. Innocent and aghast, Jean swears she loves Effie and will never marry. That, Rose snaps, "has exactly as much and as little weight as your word for it. I leave it to your conscience to estimate that wonderful amount." And she stalks off, carrying Effie toward the river dividing the two houses.

This can be great fun to read, once we accept we're not going to get quite what we came for. Scene after scene offers a quick, lustrous dazzle showered on a subject James hasn't the will to deepen with the rich resonance of meditation. Elsewhere, as he explains time and again in the Prefaces, his subject is the parade of impressions and perceptions through an individual consciousness, not the stagey events that generate them. Isabel Archer's realization of what she has made of her life, Strether's growing awareness of what he's not made of his: these are the thrills that propel *The Portrait of a Lady* and *The Ambassadors*. In *The Other House*, the refinements of character are minimal: Rose casts "a measureless white ray," "a great cold luster." The glories are sharp and snazzy, not profound. Because it was conceived as a play—and never thoroughly reimagined as a novel—we get no inner life, no nascent, intimate awareness, none of the shape and innuendo of emotion gathering and solidifying.

Instead of marking the motions of the mind, James blocks out his characters' moves. Upon learning of the death of his child, Tony:

dropped upon a bench with his wretched face in his hands, while Rose, with a passionate wail, threw herself, appalled, on the grass, and their companion, in a colder dismay, looked from one prostrate figure to the other.

The dramatic form also persists in pesky circumlocutions: "An observer of the scene would not have failed to divine . . ." Or, "Tony's face, for an initiated observer, would have shown . . ." Those "observers," or sometimes "auditors," are the vestigial audience, silent witnesses in the theater of James's mind.

All this is genius with a headache or a heartache, scattering itself with abandon: a performance worth watching. And one that exposes, more defiantly than anywhere else, a raw anarchic streak. That James violates the traditions of the murder novel by letting the crime go unpunished isn't surprising. Since when did his moral agons take place in any ordinary world of judges or juries? One arresting virtue *The Other House* insists on is making its own rules. Police or medical examiners would be out of place; James's justice is a form of elite vigilantism. There is no polity, only the clutch of characters—and a few servants to be placated with lies. In its consistency of vision, its perverse refusal to honor the conventions, *The Other House* is beautifully whole, as its author might say. And deeply unsettling—not the master we thought we knew.

In 1909, at the age of sixty-six, his great work behind him, James was once more writing plays, which says something about blind tenacity. Two of them, both based on old stories, were staged. Then he turned again to *The Other House*. Was it the abiding good husbandry of the true professional? Why let the old scenario go to waste? He managed to get a producer interested, but practical difficulties arose, and besides, James was "sickened" by the cuts and changes made to his script. Clearly he hated to let it go. Perhaps its theme, the ruthlessness that passion can lead to, wouldn't let him go. The play was never produced.

Trans Fish

It may come as a surprise to learn that we're not the only species that can undertake sex changes. And while the procedure is fairly recent with us, our distant ancestors, fish—at least certain kinds of fish—have been managing such transformations for millennia, without any of the nasty repercussions all too common among humans. For with the media's increasing coverage of sex changes, ignorance and prejudice continue to stir up ill-will and even violence against trans people.

So, in an effort to educate the public and promote social harmony, a look at how our undersea relations handle these sensitive matters is in order. Granted, the ways of fish are not always for us. Yet there is something to be learned from their unique sexual culture, which glides along tranquilly and serves the interests of the whole community. A placard on display in front of a glass case at the Maui Ocean Center in Hawaii declares, "The females of many species of fishes can become males when circumstances require it."

What are the "circumstances"? To begin with, these "many species of fish" live in harems. As in human harems, one male—the largest fish—consorts with all the females. Much as the practice may repel us, living in all-female harems has proven advantageous for fish, though I am by no means suggesting that we adopt it. According to the Maui Ocean Center, it ensures the survival of the group.

When the lord of the harem dies, he is replaced by the

largest female, who becomes a male, overnight as it were—no medications or arduous surgical procedures are required. The female simply changes sex and color; her eggs are absorbed (where and how are not specified), and she, now he, begins to produce sperm.

One obvious drawback is that the custom grants an unfair privilege to size, making it the single criterion for sexual power—happily not the case among humans, trans or not. Height may be a factor in our mating, but it is hardly the only one, or even the most important. Great lovers of the past, male or female, were not notable for height. By all accounts Cleopatra was short. So was Napoleon. In the fabled romances of myth and history—Paris and Helen, Tristan and Isolde, Abelard and Heloise, Orpheus and Eurydice—no mention is made of height.

Indeed, the female fish themselves might prefer other fishy qualities in their harem lord. Appearance, temperament, speed and grace of swimming, whatever female fish find a turn-on. Unfortunately, no relevant data on that subject is available.

A striking peculiarity of these fish societies, and the one that most distinguishes it from our own, is the absence of natural-born males. Apparently all the fish are originally female—contradicting the Biblical account: "Male and female created He them." Unlike human embryos, in which all brains begin as female and some change to male during gestation, in fish, this fundamental step is absent. Simone de Beauvoir famously writes in *The Second Sex*, "Women are not born but made." In the case of fish, it's the males who are not born but made.

(This singular aspect of fish life recalls the all-female societies that feminist writers such as Charlotte Perkins Gilman envisioned in their utopian fictions. Of course those were fantasies that could be realized only by barbarically un-acceptable measures.)

The mores of the harem guarantee that all members are able to reproduce, with all sperm and eggs entering and reviv-ifying the gene pool. "This ensures the highest reproductive capacity of each individual," according to the placard at the Maui Ocean Center. Plus everyone has a chance to enjoy an active sex life, something highly desirable in any species. "No member of the harem needs to swim around looking for a mate, and there are no small males to be pushed aside by larg-er males during mating." The opportunity to mate without raw competition or the frustrations of dating is certainly a benefit. In other words, a good time should be had by all.

This good time, though, must depend on the energies and predilections of that large and solitary male (formerly female). As in any harem, he might favor certain females and neglect others. And while the gene pool contains am-ple diversity among the female contributors, his are the only sperm. Possibly he has a short life, worn out from his fertiliz-ing duties, so that the male contribution to the gene pool is frequently refreshed.

How do the fish feel about their mode of life? As with us, there may be some females who feel misplaced in their bodies, or simply desire the prerogatives of maleness, like girls who become Little League baseball champions only to discover they're barred from the major leagues. Perhaps the largest female fish is of that persuasion. She waits impatiently for the lord of the harem to die so she can assume his role, producing sperm rather than eggs and having her way with her companions.

But what if she is content with her gender identity and has no wish to change? Must she accept her fate in a spirit of sacrifice, the way the strongest young men in ancient Greek or Aztec rites had to be sacrificed for the continued prosperity of the group? Or can she pass the questionable honor on to the second largest female, or the next in line who is willing and eager?

Other critical questions remain murky. How often does the change occur? What is a fish's normal life span and how often do they like to mate? Every few days? Once a week? All night long?

It's probable that when the change occurs, relationships in the wet harem go out of whack for a while. No community, watery or otherwise, can withstand such drastic social upheaval without showing some strain. (Witness how exercised certain of our state legislators are over the relatively trivial matter of bathroom use.) To begin with, the females are accustomed to regarding the newly trans male as a sisterly comrade. Suddenly her sex change kicks in and they must accept her as lord of the harem. Even more, they must accept her (now his) sexual attentions, which most likely start out tentative and awkward, given her (his) lack of experience in that line.

But maybe the fish are so used to their time-honored customs that they take them in stride, as it were. After all, they are fish. Maybe they have a graceful, fluid approach to it all. Maybe, unlike us, they manage these things swimmingly.

Using a Cane

For a few months after spinal surgery I needed to use a cane. Both my mother and my older sister before me had been advised to use a cane but my mother refused because she thought it made her look like an old person; she was eighty-one at the time. My sister accepted the cane but chose one—actually she bought several—with elaborate wood carvings at the handles and other striking features of color and design, canes that expressed character and taste the way her clothes or boots or umbrellas did. As long as she had to use it, she felt, she would make it part of her ensemble.

I might have done the same had I thought the cane would be permanent, but I expected to be using it for only a short while, until I had fully recovered. In fact I preferred the cane to have a nondescript, provisional look, a look that implied I was not really dependent on a cane, or only temporarily. I got the standard chrome pharmacy supplies cane, with notches along the shaft to adjust its height. The most unobtrusive cane possible.

On my first few outings with the cane, I found myself almost unwittingly trying to make eye contact with other cane users as if to establish a connection, acknowledgment of a common need, but this rarely succeeded. Apparently carrying a cane was not sufficient grounds for any personal rapport. Those who were habituated to the cane were no longer preoccupied with it, as I was.

Walking outdoors with the cane, I became a different person. An old woman with a cane. (Or "elderly," though

I've always found that euphemism worse than "old.") I felt at a disadvantage. I wanted to announce, or maybe to wear a placard saying, There's no need to pity me, I'm just like you, I work, I have a family, and besides, I'll only be needing this for a couple of months.

At the same time, the cane made me feel distinctive, the bearer of a mystery. Why on earth was someone who looked healthy and active using a cane? I had occasionally wondered that about cane carriers, but only in passing, without any genuine interest. Why should anyone wonder about me? But I suppose we all tend to believe we are more noticed by strangers than we truly are. Often when I feel observed, I have to remind myself that strangers are surely mulling over their own affairs, as complicated and absorbing to them as mine are to me.

Not only did I feel different, but I was regarded differently by the caneless, who opened doors for me, stepped out of my path, generally showed small courtesies. I enjoyed that. I like having things done for me so I needn't exert myself. (I do pick up things dropped nearby by old people or pregnant women.) Even before my cane, I always acceded when men held the door open for me though it contradicted my principles. Inertia trumped principles.

When people I knew in the neighborhood stopped to ask what happened—why the cane?—I was more than happy to tell the story of my surgery. But I tried to be brief so I didn't become a bore on the subject of "my operation." On the other hand, when people I knew equally well ignored the cane, I felt frustrated, misperceived: they must think I've gotten old and frail enough to need a cane. I longed to tell them that was not the case.

Drivers behaved so much better. Cars making turns stopped and waited while I walked slowly across their path.

Taxis, usually very aggressive in New York City, slowed down so I could pass. I took my time, enjoying my privilege. Whereas before the cane, I tended to hurry along when I was delaying waiting cars, now I had no qualms about making them wait. No one could blame a person with a cane for walking slowly.

Right around when I started using the cane, I began a tutorial with a student in the narrative medicine program at Columbia University, a doctor who needed help writing her thesis. The very first day she came over, I met her at the door with my cane and preceded her down the hall. She immediately told me I was using the cane wrong. I didn't know there was a right and wrong way to use a cane—it seemed the simplest of devices, even for the mechanically challenged. She said I had to hold the cane opposite to my weaker side—the side more affected by the surgery—and set it down together with the foot of that side. This was hard to get used to but it certainly felt better.

With my cane firmly on the proper side—the left—I began noticing many things I'd never noticed before. The first was how many people carried canes. All at once cane-users appeared to swarm through my neighborhood. Some were old or bent over or disabled in some way, or a combination of all three. Some walked peculiarly even with the aid of a cane, recalling the classic Monty Python sketch, "The Ministry of Silly Walks." A number of canes had an extra section at the bottom with four little feet for greater stability.

Other cane users were not old and looked to be in good shape (as I hoped I did), and a few moved along at quite an impressive clip, far beyond my powers. What could be their problem? Here and there I spied the smart-looking canes with the fancy carvings, but far more common was the plain functional cane like mine. Perhaps those people, too, were temporary cane-users, or else they didn't care what impression they made on the street, or didn't consider the cane part of their presentation of self in public life, to borrow the sociologist Erving Goffman's felicitous phrase.

I also became more aware of people with crutches. Even before my cane days I had noticed people on crutches, either the old-fashioned wooden kind—now nearly extinct—or the newer chrome kind with circular metal loops for the arms. I was sympathetic. But with cane in hand, I felt a twinge of superiority to the crutch people: You're worse off than I, in a different category entirely, was my ungenerous response. I need only a cane, and temporarily at that. You're on crutches, maybe forever.

Once I felt confident enough after my surgery to attempt the New York City subways, the cane became a magic wand. The instant I entered a crowded subway car, someone would get up to give me a seat. I didn't even have to wave it around. Formerly, I would occasionally be offered a seat by younger people. Maybe half the time. With the cane my record was one hundred percent of the time. If my husband or a friend around my age happened to be with me, they were frequently offered a seat next to me, the second person inspired by the sacrifice of the first. For two and a half months I never lacked for a seat on the subway. Afterward, it was not easy to get accustomed to standing again. I missed the cane and its magic powers. Now I wanted to announce or wear a placard saying: I just recently stopped using a cane, how about giving me a seat?

At last I decided it was time to wean myself from the cane. I would carry it with me but use it intermittently. A block with, a block without. This proved a good regimen. However, on the alternate blocks when I carried the cane on my arm, I wondered what people were thinking. Why is she carrying a cane if she's not using it? Maybe she's bringing it to a friend. Again, I knew no one would care, but I liked imagining myself an object of curiosity, objectifying myself. I would have liked to proclaim, or to wear a placard saying, I'm getting used to walking without the cane, one block on one block off . . .

Soon I started forgetting the cane when I went out, leaving it hooked on a dining room chair, its accustomed place. The first time I forgot it, already out the door and on the street, I decided to do without it, but after a couple of blocks, walking became uncomfortable—I wasn't ready to go cane-less. I had to go back for it.

Then there came a time when I barely noticed I'd forgotten it. That was when I realized the era of the cane, its privileges and drawbacks, was over. I could stop thinking about it and resume thinking about whatever I used to think about while walking down the street. Whatever that was.

First Loves

At age six, there was Bradley with freckles and a voice oddly raspy for his age, the same as mine. A witty boy who laughed a lot; his freckles glowed with humor. We walked to school together holding hands. He grew up to manage a Las Vegas casino and, as rumor had it, dealt drugs on the side. Not suitable at all for the long haul. I can see us hand in hand, walking down East New York Avenue, looking both ways at every corner, finally making it to the schoolyard and running to our respective lines. This was true love. Our romance was brief, but all the years through high school, when we met in the halls, we greeted each other warmly, ripples of memory passing between us.

The next was a girl, Paula. I was nine. It was her name that drew me, exotic, so different from the names of my daily friends, the Barbaras, Carols, Judys and Susans of Brooklyn. Paula came from afar, somewhere upstate, and visited her aunt and uncle across the street during school vacations. Distance, too, was exotic. There was little distance in Brooklyn, the outer or inner sort. I always craved the exotic; my father mocked me when I used the word. Also exotic was Paula's skin, not black, that wouldn't have been possible on our block back then, but brown like a Native American or a Mexican although she was neither, most likely descended from Sephardic Jews of the Middle East. I waited eagerly for my mother to announce, Paula's here. I rushed across the street to ring her bell. I didn't know then that I was in love.

I picture her sitting on my bed, both of us cross-legged,

playing cards or playing with dolls or simply talking about whatever nine-year-olds talk about. After a year or so, she stopped coming. Paula, wherever you are, I missed you so.

Thirteen, a bad year for any girl. We summered in the Catskills, a site of torpor worse even than Brooklyn, and shared a wall and porch with the family next door. The two sons, sixteen and nineteen, worked in the day camp. It was the older boy I mooned over, as girls often fix on the unattainable. He was large and dark (dark like Paula), with black hair in a crew cut, a handsome beefy face, good-natured, unmarred by thought or introspection. He walked around in bathing trunks, making it easy for me to admire his tanned body and hairy legs. For some forgotten reason he called me Tex; I thrilled to the name. One day I sat on my porch in my bathing suit, holding my towel, hoping he would appear. And, miracle, his screen door opened and out he came in his trunks, carrying a towel. Hi, Tex. His voice sliced a path through my innards. I remember the slicing feeling to this day. Going to the pool? I nodded. Me too, he said. Walk with me. Indescribable joy, walking down the dirt road with Lenny, hoping ardently that my friends would see us. It was almost like a date. I dreamed that from then on we'd be a couple, like the many transient couples the summer shaped—only coupledom could ease the smothering dullness—those little loves that ended at Labor Day. But when we reached the pool, he joined his friends and I joined mine. I'd been imagining some horseplay in the water, maybe with a ball.

I relived that five-minute walk all through the summer and the deadly fall. Some years later I married a boy, not my preferred dark or brawny. I loved him anyway. I imagined he was taller than he was. We talked on the phone at night for hours, I in my older sister's bedroom I'd inherited when she left to get married, as every girl had to do. I was amazed to find a boy who could actually talk and who read books. I didn't realize till later that such boys were plentiful if you had the patience to wait and knew where to look. It was like buying the first house that you see, and sometimes that works out quite well. I love him but as we grow old I wonder how I could have plunged so thoughtlessly, blind-eyed, into the future with a stranger.

Beyond the Garden

He knew he wanted to taste that fruit as badly as she did. On his own, he would have come round to it in time, despite his father's obdurate command. But since her arrival he had lost the habit of fetching his own food. She always shared whatever fruits she gathered, so it became natural in him to wait. Besides, he enjoyed watching her climb the trees. Very possibly, he admitted in the privacy of his heart, he had been waiting for that very fruit.

So from the moment he betrayed her to his father—the thundering, awesome voice that must come from an equally awesome shape, or shapelessness—he felt slightly ashamed, a new and unwelcome feeling. Ashamed not of the eating but of the telling. Of course his father would have found out (he knew everything yet seemed to relish humiliating him by questions), but there wouldn't have been that shifty guilt each time he looked at her or touched her, a guilt more particular than the encompassing guilt he felt in the presence of the voice. And she certainly didn't make things any easier: docile acceptance was not in her nature, in the beginning, at any rate. She railed and stormed about loyalty, and said being a helpmeet worked both ways, he utterly failed to understand her being with him and all that it implied. . . . Like his father, she had words at her command, piercingly direct words, and the more she spoke, the worse he felt.

Well, let her complain. There were things she couldn't begin to appreciate. What it was to have such a father, for one. How would she like to have awakened, all alone, to the sound of a voice that shook your insides? A voice that wouldn't for a moment let you forget that whatever you used and enjoyed came from his power and at his pleasure. Another thing: while it was abundantly clear where she came from—you'd think a man might sleep undisturbed and call his body his own—his ambiguous origin made him uneasy. That the voice was his father, everything's father, he had no choice but to take on faith. Yet he was told, too, that he came from a handful of dust. That was far from reassuring. At the moments of his greatest strength, when he sported with the animals or swam across the stream, he would suddenly think, dust, and shiver with visions of crumbling, dissolving. And could she feel what a burden it was to live up to his father's image? For those were the cryptic words he must live by—made in his image—yet how could a creature of dust aspire to such grandeur?

None of this meant a thing to her. In her view, he worried far too much over his relation to his father. Why not concentrate instead on his relation to her, a notion that struck him as sacrilege. She just wasn't important enough in the scheme of things, delightful as it might be to play with her and end up, more often than not, in an embrace. Did his father indulge in such lush pleasures? Inconceivable. It was one thing to yield briefly, and quite another to take it seriously: hardly in that sober image.

So he had obeyed the voice and told the truth, as he was taught to do (threats being his father's way of teaching), and they were cast out of the garden to a colder, craggier place, where he could never hear the voice approach without trembling. They were poor, as warned, but the work did not trouble him—indeed, the idleness of the garden had become tedious. He suspected he was made for more than leisure, that he had the resources to achieve something, to make something. Look what his father had made in a mere seven days. If work was his curse, he was ready to endure it.

He didn't grasp the nature of her curse until he saw it. This was no curse but a blessing. Of all the stupendous things, of all the examples of his father's inventiveness, this was the most miraculous. She heaved and moaned and wailed while he, standing helplessly by, thought at first that it must be Death, that baffling, dread word. At last, out of all her heaving, came another exactly like him. Her wails stopped immediately and they both laughed in astonished joy.

But why, he couldn't help wondering after the shock had passed, had his father given this great power to her? Was she the preferred one? Was it because he was made of dust and she of firmer stuff? As for the child, it had what neither of them had ever known, a mother. His own child was more privileged than he, motherless dust. All he had were his strength and will to work.

The next year there was another like him. The others were like her, and less startling, after the first. Besides, they seemed to belong more to her than to him, what with her carrying and nursing and tending them while he was at work. He could feel her gradually turning away from him and toward them. She still came when he wanted her, but not with exclusive devotion. And just as these thoughts came to trouble him, the terrible thing happened between the boys.

It was he who discovered them, and who heard the older one saying those rash, unforgivable words to the great voice, which thundered more terrifyingly than when it had cast them from the garden years ago. When it finally withdrew, leaving him to gaze at his sons, the one defiant, confused, and ashamed, the other a mangled body on the grass, he understood he had lost them both forever. Death was no longer a mere word.

He mourned and cursed life. Her grief was inconsolable. Once so lavish with words, now she had none. This was beyond her imagining. The life oozed out of her as it had out of the boy, though she still breathed and moved. She aged overnight. She lost interest in everything, even in him.

No one remained but his daughters, who looked almost as she had done when she first appeared. Up to this moment he had regarded them simply as tender children to care for, who could help with the work when they grew strong enough. Now, with discomfort, he watched as they moved through the house or the fields, precisely as he had once watched her, bewitched by every nuance of contour and movement. Would it be so very wrong? It was nothing his father had specifically forbidden.

In time he bred a long line of sons and daughters. They were fruitful and multiplied, as commanded. To his growing horror, their vices multiplied with their numbers. After Eve's shock at the first brutal act, none of it surprised her much. She observed with mute disapproval. Her silence plagued him, and her occasional yielding to him was diffident. Her silence cast a pall over the projects absorbing his every waking hour. For his talent, he had discovered, was for invention: he made machines—massive and powerful, delicate and intricate—which could perform feats never dreamed of in the garden. Perhaps even his father had never dreamed of them, though that was hard to say. He was no longer in close touch with his father, speaking to him only when unavoidable, and in a perfunctory way. His father was apparently content to do the same, and his voice seemed to come from farther off than before.

The machines could control the elements, channel water and cut through rock and tear through sky. They were his delight; they swelled his pride. With certain fine instruments he solved the enigmas of his own body. He learned that she had not accomplished that first miracle, ages back, on her own. She could never have done it without him. This was deeply satisfying. He had created something animate; he was made in his father's image, after all.

As time unreeled, he treated her as his father had treated him. Living up to the image, I see, she noted with a touch of irony. Sometimes she rebelled, sometimes she acquiesced. She was exploring her powers too, and no longer preoccupied with him alone.

Peace and plenty were hard to come by, and life was full of difficulties. The garden was long gone, a dimming sweet memory. They fell into a pattern, an unspoken arrangement to keep the peace, and keep the passion as well. They accepted that between them would forever be a shifting, tilting, perilous balance that tipped one way or the other at the slightest stirring of the air. And so it continued, from light to night and back again, until time reeled out its last seconds, leaving only the void.

Only Connect

I've lost count of how many articles I've read lately offering sympathy and therapeutic remedies to addicts who cannot detach from their cell phones. Their addiction is not to the phone's original purpose, human connection, which might not be so bad. No, people are talking on the phone less than ever, I'm told by those in the know. It's the rest of it, the whole world miniaturized and embedded in the back pockets of their jeans, when not at the ear.

Primitive cell phones used to make me laugh: people ambled down the street alone, chattering or arguing. I dismissed them as run-of-the-mill lunatics. Now the phones are as essential as keys or wallets, and like therapy dogs, they can be taken anywhere. It's not considered rude to whip one out during a family gathering, a tête-à-tête, and maybe even on more intimate occasions. And there's that discouraging sight of couples in a restaurant, each busy on their phones.

Like everyone else, I possess a cell phone, but I have no fondness for it. I don't hold it at all times and don't give out the number. The calls I miss are in a foreign language, or from robotic voices, or wrong numbers. I resent it because it has superseded the real phone, with which I had a long, close, and affectionate relationship beginning in infancy. Whenever the phone rang, I toddled to answer, but it was soon grabbed away by some hovering adult.

Later, in the seventh grade, tall, erect Miss Mulcare introduced me to the nuances of telephone etiquette. Lesson one: Never phone a friend and say, "Hello, is Claudia there?"

Instead say, "This is Lynne. May I please speak to Claudia?" If we knew the parent answering, we must say, "Hello, Mrs. Jones. This is Lynne," and perhaps even add, "How are you?" depending on our degree of acquaintance and of aplomb.

Miss Mulcare was austere, and with age the rosy skin of her face had grown softly tufted, like certain pillows. Her hair was speckled gray and white. We, her students, were smooth of cheek, young enough to remember the aura of power and privilege attaching to the phone, the infantile thrill of finally being allowed to burble a few words and hear, magically, an answering voice.

We had phone privileges now, but they came with obligations. Lesson two from Miss Mulcare: Never open with, "Who is this?" The caller, the invader of privacy, rather than the callee, must declare herself. The phone was an intrusion, maybe a summons, and the person intruded upon or summoned was entitled, at the very least, to a smidgen of courtesy. To this day I'm appalled by callers who, not having had the benefit of Miss Mulcare, open crudely with "Is John there?"

The phone offered adventures in automation. I loved to dial the numbers that gave the time (with the fitting exchange of Meridian) or the weather report. How thrilling to hold the receiver without uttering a word and hear: "At the tone, the time will be . . . one forty-five a.m." There couldn't be a woman, could there, sitting by the phone day and night repeating that sentence? No, I could sense a shift in the air, a hollowness, before the time was announced, so that even then I knew it was a recording that would play till the crack of doom with only the number alive and changing, just as the moments on a wall clock tick by unvaryingly, but the lived quality of each moment has a fresh taste and texture. The weather report was fun too: without saying a word you were forewarned, though with meteorological science in its salad days, the predictions were nowhere near so accurate as they are today.

My adolescent friends and I could talk on the phone endlessly (as today kids text), even if we would be meeting in school the following morning. Most households had only one phone, so parents were continually warning us not to "tie up the phone," an early instance of FOMO.

The accoutrements and scope of the phone evolved drastically through my childhood and young adulthood. Gone are the comic movie scenes of rows of seated operators jabbing wires into switchboards, operators whose antic garbling of messages drove the helter-skelter plot. They were replaced by answering services, used by those who couldn't afford to miss a call—doctors, actors waiting for a callback, and those troubled by the ever-present FOMO.

In old movies, or new movies and TV shows set in olden times, we get a glimpse of primitive phones used in a cute, self-conscious manner, such as the telephone that entered the lives of the younger generation in the televised version of Galsworthy's *Forsyte Saga*. Or the telephone in the TV series *Upstairs, Downstairs*, handled with cautious deference by the impeccable butler, Hudson. These phones were clumsy affairs, a tubular receiver and a boxlike speaker on the wall into which the characters shout: sweet campy objects that make us grin. The Forsytes never treated their phone casually: if it rang, both they and we knew something noteworthy was afoot. As I watch many of the old films, when critical situations demand speedy reactions, I find myself thinking, Oh, if only they had a cell phone.

One of the first jarring signs that automation was afoot was the loss of our beautiful and evocative exchanges, our Butterfields, our Murray Hills, our Morningsides. Obliterated overnight and replaced by digits. One may not feel attached to a social security number or a zip code, but Plaza, Riverside, and Chelsea were no mere clues to location. They were charmed possessions, tokens of identity. Trafalgar, Cloverdale, and Esplanade conferred their multisyllabic glamour on us, but there is no glamour to living in the 468 neighborhood. Numbers do have their own evocative symbolism—the monotheistic solidity of 1 or the Christian triad of 3, or the satanic connotations of 6—but will never have the poetry of letters, which make names and conjure association and memory. We accepted the deprivation meekly; we were taken aback, unprepared. We should have fought for our exchanges, kept using them defiantly. A handful of numbers in my address book are still listed by their exchanges—sweet nostalgias, bitter reminders.

In those days of Axminster, Baring, and Shore Road, my parents' friends would unexpectedly ring the doorbell—"We were just passing by"—and be invited in for coffee. The hour might be inopportune, but these were friends, after all, and they were made welcome. Social meetings nowadays are scheduled in advance; doorbells are silent but phones clamor. Or you're settling into the tub after worrying all day about a loved one in trouble. What will the blood tests reveal? Will he get the job he needs so badly? The phone rings. Never mind the machine: love propels you, dripping, toward the news. Hello? You pant. It's Planned Parenthood and they need your help.

Everyone needs our help. The causes are worthy and the callers are shameless, but try as they may to sound friendly, the voices give them away: unctuous, bright, a tad edgy, prepared for your hostility. They read from scripts, greet you by name. They have the audacity to ask, "How are you this evening?" as if it mattered.

Hanging up is the best solution. But hanging up, like

breaking up, is hard to do—like slamming the door in some-one's face. I know overly courteous people who'll hear out the whole script before saying no. (Though these calls have their occasional uses. A recently divorced friend developed a warm long-distance relationship with a charming real estate salesman. Good practice for real life, no strings attached. She enjoyed the distraction and solicitude, along with the power to say no endlessly without discouraging her suitor.)

Next came the calls from no one—a mere voice. You are the winner of a three-foot rubber raft, suitable for water sports. Or, Sorry I missed you. I'm running for office and I'd like you to vote for me. Those virtual sentences jar our notions of what qualifies as talk.

"Reach out and touch someone" was the slogan of an old AT&T advertising campaign. The aim of the personal call was to arrange a meeting. The conversation itself might cover every topic under the sun, even ascend—or descend—to intimacy. Still it was only a prelude, a snatch of delights to come if we signed on for the full experience, like a trailer for a movie. In time, though, the phone call became the visit, as though nothing essential or significant would be added were the speakers to meet. Physical presence, the sensory aware-ness of others, came to count for little. The phone call as a form of social life—or the phone visit, perhaps arranged by appointment—is related to minimalism and conceptual art, which came about around the same time, and in which bare allusions are acceptable substitutes for the real thing.

During the pandemic, phone conversations enjoyed something of a revival—we needed each other. Though not quite an art form, they were evolving in that direction. We might have ended up labeling people as good on the phone, just as we call them good company or good listeners or good dancers or good in bed. In fact I label them so already. There were moments—especially during the period of isolation—when nothing would serve so well as a long chummy talk, curled up in a chair, analyzing the day's events with an absurd yet exhilarating minuteness. I sought out friends who blossomed on the phone. I could feel them settling in, summoning their resources of clarity and empathy, calling forth my own best flights too.

Conversely, with friends who live too far away for a visit, we talk so well and so thoroughly on the phone that we don't ever long to see them. If they do hit town periodically, we feel a discrepancy, a slight jolt when we meet in person. We're so accustomed to the unfleshed voice that we have trouble compounding it with the body it issues from. By the time our neural circuits have wedded the voice and the body, the visit may be over, the critical moment passed. We go home unsatisfied, looking forward to the next phone call, as if we haven't really been with the friend we know so well. Something was missing: an absence, the fertile vacuum in which our friendship flourished.

If certain friendships are best cultivated over the phone, certain things are more easily said too. Asking favors is easier over the phone. So is refusing them, especially for those who find it hard to say no; the phone removes the guilt-inducing sight of the other's disappointment. Anger, a sharper way of saying no, is also easier over the phone, at least for the timid, who can hang up when the rising temperature begins crackling the wires. (The brave and belligerent may relish the heat of confrontation.) The timid, again, profit by the phone, for instance when encountering someone in a position of power, say, a prospective employer. They can sit quaking and unkempt in their bathrobes, heedless of facial expressions, gestures and all the rest. Apologizing is easier over the phone, though without the sight of a forgiving face, one tends to apologize for too long, trying to make the forgiveness palpable. A telephone encounter is a great equalizer for those who for one reason or another feel unpresentable. Still, none of this helps if you're phonophobic, an ailment more widespread than is generally recognized; it may soon have its flurry of media attention and support groups, in which phoning fellow sufferers will be the first step in recovery.

Finally, saying goodbye is easier over the phone.

Easier to avoid the emotion that attends direct experience. One of phone culture's many results—good or bad, depending on your outlook—is to dilute strong emotion, often to the vanishing point. To make everything personal feel, to some degree, like business. The phone makes us businesslike; it makes us conduct our lives like cottage industries, with appointments, calendar juggling, quick jotting of memos, names and numbers.

In the world of business there are no interruptions. Or rather, interruption *means* business—action, transaction, goods and money flowing. A business with silent phones is on the path to doom. So with our lives, we want the phone to ring. It means we have a life, we're in business. And the ways we conduct our little businesses—from hello to goodbye—illustrate what the late social philosopher Erving Goffman so aptly termed the presentation of self in everyday life.

Some defensive people feel they must greet the world with a steely formality. They pick up with an officious, off-putting "Hello," and then, if it's a friend, relax immediately into a colloquial tone. I've been told my "Hello" sounds a world-weary, "What now?" note—if not expecting the worst, then at least something pretty bad. This doesn't surprise me. Our every gesture shows how we anticipate that the world will impinge on us—for impinge it must, even in the safety of home, assaulting the open gate of the ear. The world's approach, for me, is an interruption of the inner dialogue, at once fantastical and mundane, in which I'm usually absorbed. The intruding call has about as much charm as a stranger bursting in on a rendezvous. I wouldn't want to be greeted by a "Hello" like mine, and luckily I'm not. The great majority, whose comfort in the universe I can barely imagine, pick up with a tone of merry preparedness: what delightful new event is about to befall me?

Endings tell as much as beginnings. The conversation draws to its natural close, but some people cherish the long goodbye. Either they dread the silence awaiting them or they cannot stop whatever they're doing, whether pleasant or painful. The longer they've been doing it, the harder it is to switch gears. A long conversation becomes incrementally longer, like the drawn-out conclusion of a Romantic symphony. I'm usually restless to return to the inner dialogue once the end is in sight. I begin to hang up, but a dimming voice comes wistfully from the lowered receiver. "Sorry, what was that?" Nothing, usually. Except in cases where the speaker leaves the crucial item, the real purpose of the call, for last—"I forgot to mention, I'm getting married and moving to Spain."

Suitable hours for calling were a key feature of Miss Mulcare's phone etiquette. Perhaps she began her career in a hospital or reform school, for she warned us never to call anyone past nine o'clock in the evening. Life in general seemed to take place earlier back then; whenever the phone rang at ten-thirty at night, my mother, yawning over her two-cents-a-day rental novel, would groan wearily, "There's Uncle George again," as if he were violating a curfew. (She had a near-infallible phone instinct, a kind of sonic ESP. "That's your sister," she'd inform my father at the first ring. Or, "Oh, good, it's the plumber," and she was usually correct.)

The disparity in phoning hours points up what far-apart galaxies we inhabit. Lots of callers feel that eight a.m., a brutal hour for talking, opens the official phoning day. And I must pick up, for what but disaster could seek me out so early? "So sorry, did I wake you?" they address my sleep-clogged voice. You're supposed to say, "Oh no, it's quite all right." But it's not all right. I'm still tangled in dreams, while they've dressed and had their coffee; their every cell is alert, carrying forward the affairs of the world.

Calls during working hours are problematic. Because the flow of work in offices, stores and elsewhere is unpredictable and sporadic, businesses claim their employees' entire days, as in the age of indentured servitude. Friends may hesitate to interrupt. Yet often there's nothing to do at work except read, write letters, take care of personal business (on the phone), and generally try to appear occupied. Personal calls may be more than welcome.

For people who work at home, the situation is different. Until the pandemic closed down so many offices, most people didn't believe anyone working at home was really working; friends had no qualms about calling. They're even doing us a favor, or so they think, bringing welcome diversion. And though I hate to expose a well-kept secret, they're not far wrong. Our first indignant thought on hearing the ring is, "Don't they know I'm working?" The next instant, reaching out eagerly: "Thank God I can stop working for a while."

The invention that changed our phone lives most dramatically was the answering machine, and I confess that this, contrary to most innovations, I have come to cherish. We wonder how we managed without it, yet manage we did. We lived more patiently. We had, perforce, the capacity to wait. But machines shape our nature as much as anything else does; this is clear by the development of phone messages, not to mention by our responses.

The messages that greet callers are another Goffman-esque presentation of self. Early messages had a naïve transparency, as in any new craft or art; in hindsight they seem touchingly ingenuous, like the great primitive paintings. Some were self-conscious, others gracious—"I'm so sorry I can't get to the phone," or as one friend archly put it, "I'm sorry to greet you with a recorded announcement." One of my favorites, showing a rare existential precision, declared, "This is the voice of John Smith."

How quickly we moved beyond all that. We're sophisticated, adaptable, ready to explore the possibilities of the form. Greetings range from friendly and functional to bare-bones terse: one close friend simply states her phone number—the ultimate in Mondrianesque. I get the point, yet I feel a chill through my bones. Must she be quite so stark? It's me! In the middle of the spectrum are the playful—snatches of popular songs hinting at the greeter's current mood, the most famous bars of Handel's "Hallelujah Chorus," homilies from Ecclesiastes or enshrined poetry, and what can only be called kitsch: the family's youngest member piping out a rehearsed sentence, sometimes assisted by a pet.

What a jolt it was, hearing my very first machine greeting. What was this eerie artifice, this absent presence? Did it actually expect me to say something in return? I was so boggled by the process that I just hung up. Later I was told that hanging up mute is a form of rudeness. How could you be rude to a machine? But evidently you could. I wonder what Miss Mulcare would have thought of that: machines expecting all the courtesy due to their owners.

I made judgments of character, in those frontier days,

based on who had answering machines. But as they proliferated like kudzu, my categories broke down. It was not merely the trendy or the self-important, but just plain folk. A select few, I thought, would never succumb: too old-fashioned, too independent, temperamentally ill-suited. How wrong I was. In the end, in an upheaval that changed the nature of personal connection, everyone succumbed.

Our styles of responding to a machine are as varied as our voices themselves. Most callers keep their usual speech patterns and personalities. But a few are curiously altered, the kindly becoming imperious, the reserved loquacious. Romantic, volatile souls turn lucid and precise, and vice versa. Who can say why? Gone are the amateur days of fumble and stammer. We're prepared for the canned greeting. We talk freely, maybe even more freely than had we reached an actual person. Indeed, sometimes we prefer to reach a machine and are startled by a real voice—Oh, I didn't think you'd be home, we stammer. And we're inhibited, as once we were inhibited by the machine; we need to revise our planned speech to make it fit for live consumption.

Spartan callers wouldn't dream of confiding anything to a machine; they leave austere names and numbers, sending us scurrying for a pencil. Their opposites address my recorded voice as if it were my receptive presence, telling it everything they would tell me. I sit down to listen, chuckling or frowning as I would at any amazingly lifelike performance. I'm in no hurry to call back; it seems I've already had the zesty human exchange, and in so undemanding a fashion too.

As a rule I return calls promptly and willingly. But not always. The machine, with its demand for a response, makes the nuances of connection pitilessly explicit. We can gauge our feelings for people by how soon we find ourselves calling back and by the vigor we bring to the task. Even worse, our caller can do the same. So we are fated to discover the degree of our own attachments, as well as how keenly others feel attached to us.

Until fairly recently it wasn't uncommon to ignore a ringing phone, provided you didn't have aged parents or young children on the loose. It was an impersonal act, or personal in the deepest sense—an assertion that privacy matters, that the uninterrupted flow of consciousness is our true life, maybe our only entitlement. But even if we have the strength of character to let the phone ring, the gesture is no longer the same. What was once a refusal has become a mere deferral. The answering machine will take the call. And as we all know, standing by while a plaintive voice addresses our machine makes us feel not private but roguishly perverse—a perverseness tinged with an unsavory sense of power.

The many new technological wonders of the phone call—Call Forwarding, Call Waiting, Redial and all the rest—magnify unsightly fault lines in human nature, although with the cell phone ubiquitous, they are used less. There's something authoritative about a ringing phone, and the new devices encourage us to leap like good soldiers to the sound of authority. Even more, they appeal to latent desperation, the sore need to feel connected. How, they hint, can we afford to miss news that might change our lives? They suggest that our present lives are not quite enough, not quite right. And existentially speaking, that may well be. Insufficiency and imperfection are built into the human condition and are the impetus for art and science, love and crime. But they will not be remedied, or at least only temporarily, by a phone call.

One salient result of the new phone technology is that the sound of the busy signal is heard no more in the land. The busy signal has been laid to rest without the proper obsequies. Brought down by what a 1994 *New York Times* article calls, "the demands of a frenetic society that increasingly sees the busy signal as a symbol of failure and lost opportunity, a vestige of the past that is no longer tolerable." Lost opportunity? Symbol of failure? Harsh words. The busy signal could be irksome, yes, but it was reassuring too. The object of desire was nearly within our grasp—tantalizingly there but not there. The preconditions of story, of romance. A little while longer and our efforts would be rewarded. Just as uncertainty gives ordinary life the fine edge of suspense, the chance of a busy signal added tension to the banal act of phoning. Now, with the phone machine, Call Redial, and so on, there's almost always success, of some sort or other. These semi-successes offer a restless semi-satisfaction which, as with sex, food, and sleep, is arguably worse than none at all.

If the busy signal has not been suitably mourned, its boorish stand-in, Call Waiting, has been too naïvely welcomed, like the stranger of legend who knocks on the door in a storm and is given a place by the hearth, then makes off with the family heirlooms. Call Waiting feeds the basest of impulses—greed and opportunism. It plays on the nasty little need to know what or who might be better than what we've got now. More than a need: again a fear, judging by the Pavlovian alacrity with which people respond to the click, of missing out on something better. The chance of a lifetime? Or an exciting emergency that requires our attention?

For the interrupted caller, Call Waiting means being swiftly weighed in the balance. Can you compete with the allure of the unknown caller in the waiting room? If not, you must accept the rudeness that is no longer considered rudeness. (So sorry, a subsequent engagement, as Oscar Wilde prophetically said.) The busy signal avoided such little abrasions to the spirit.

Whatever role we play in the unholy Call Waiting triad, we talk on tenterhooks. Competition, judgment and impending interruption hover over our words. The exchange is vitiated, the implicit premise of undivided attention is gone. A similar form of control comes with Caller ID. Sure, Caller ID is useful in avoiding solicitations, heavy breathers and dirty talkers, as well as children playing phone games: as kids, we'd call the local funeral parlor just for the joy of saying, "I'm dying to give you my business." But the gift of control has its downside. Never again can we be sure whether our own unanswered call means no one's home or we're being rejected. Besides sowing the seeds of doubt, Caller ID spoils the surprise of a phone call. The ring may be intrusive, yet it can't help but set off a tiny thrill. Someone wants us. Who can it be? And for what? We need all the thrills we can get in this life. Grant us our shiver of suspense.

Like entropy, technical ingenuity is unstoppable. The impish new options, embraced not wisely but too well, are here to stay, and already their effects on social life are being felt. Call Forwarding, for example, ensures that your caller doesn't know where you are. He imagines you harmless at home while you're at the racetrack or in a hotel room. Marriages remain intact—a contribution to family values. A boost for privacy, at any rate. Not so Redial. Was your daughter talking to the boy you warned her off? Your son hobnobbing with his drug dealer?

I dreaded the inevitable day when we would see and be seen over the phone, and it has arrived. FaceTime offers a rare intimacy, a "come as you are" party. And again, during the pandemic it was a way to warm our solitude, seeing beloved faces, almost near enough to reach out and touch. On the other hand, one advantage of the simpler phone was that we couldn't be seen. No longer can I answer half-dressed, or hunt for lost objects, check the contents of the fridge or scribble shopping lists, and do things better accomplished in private.

Notwithstanding all this, I confess I have great affection for one clever phone game: the Conference Call. Conference Calls are festive—a regular little party, only you don't have to stand on your feet balancing drinks and paper plates, or worry that your skirt is too short or your hair frizzing up in a crowded room. Conference Calls make you feel important. They must be set up in advance; your convenience is considered. They arrive promptly. The operators are polite—they, too, must think we're important. The whole process is amiably civil. "Are you there, Lynne? Good. We've already got Bob on the line. Please hold as we get Sue and Jim and Carol. . . . Are you there, Sue? Please hold as . . . " While you wait for the others to be lassoed into the auditory corral, you can chat with the early arrivals, the kind of spontaneous free-wheeling talk of people off on a giddy spree. Suddenly a new voice is heard. Welcome, Jim. Hi, Carol. The operator, like a suave maître d', bows out and the fete can begin. The habits of group meetings shift slightly, toward the democratic. The shy are encouraged to speak, for when a voice is the sole sign of our presence, an absent voice is notable. Those who talk too much are cut off more readily than if they loomed two feet away. Time is money, so matters are settled nimbly, without awkward silences or show-offy wrangling. No travel time is involved.

Finally there is Voice Mail, the dread labyrinth; I shudder to think of Miss Mulcare ensnared in it. Whether its architects knew it or not, Voice Mail has an august history. It derives from no less than Plato, who in his *Dialogues* used a process of dichotomizing and categorizing to generate the endlessly forking, ramifying answers to philosophical questions. Centuries later the Neoplatonist scholar, Porphyry, drew so clear a branching diagram of the method that it became known as a Tree of Porphyry.

Voice Mail has reshaped our handling of daily trivia. We once relied on anonymous voices to help us dispatch life's errands. Well, no more. Voice Mail may be saving time for the corporate staff, but not the humble caller. Hearing the relentless options drone by might be borne if you could trust that eventually a category would turn up that suits your need. But it doesn't. Your need doesn't merit a slot. You wait for the human option, but all too often it doesn't exist.

Voice Mail is our latter-day Castle. Were Kafka alive, he would write a story about it: *The Phone Call*, or more likely *The Phone Kall*, and the call would never go through. Like all evil empires, it thrives by defining and restricting the choices of the citizenry. The authoritarian spirit serves only itself, setting the terms of discourse and proscribing the dialogue. It shuns the ragged edges of the unclassifiable. It renders its victims impotent and passive, ensuring that there's no human exchange.

Incidentally, if technology aims to make human contact superfluous, it had better be planning alternate arrangements for procreation: phone sex can't yet go that far. Phone sex is certainly safe sex, as well as another way of avoiding real contact. Not that it's brand-new. It's probably been around ever since phones themselves, the crucial difference being that those who were so inclined were not strangers engaged in a commercial transaction. Rather, they used the phone as a stopgap measure when they couldn't meet. Or sought diversion. (I can't picture the Forsytes or Hudson indulging, though, and as for Miss Mulcare, perish the thought.) I haven't investigated commercial phone sex, partly out of inhibition but mostly because I have a feeling it would lead to junk mail and robocalls. Anyway, if I must have sex without another person present, I prefer to have it with a book.

Making a long-distance call, now ancient history, was once a major procedure, undertaken only in unusual circumstances—dire news or grand news. It meant placing yourself in the hands of a long-distance operator, specially trained like an intensive-care nurse, who appreciated the gravity of the act. She would patiently ask for data and offer a choice of treatment—collect, or the more elite person-to-person.

Depending on your temperament, getting a long-distance call was cause for either alarm or joy. (In my childhood household it was alarm. "Long Distance calling. I have a call from so-and-so. Will you accept the charges?" My mother turned pale as she breathed an assent.) Apart from announcements of death or disaster, though, long-distance calls were a brief exotic treat, like some delicate morsel. And suitably expensive. You made sure to savor every mouthful. A modest helping might be even better than a large, lest the richness begin to cloy. That unique flavor seeped away, of course, with the advent of direct dialing. At first it was a small miracle— getting through all alone, no operator required! But very quickly it became commonplace.

Not yet so commonplace is the international call, the only phone experience that can duplicate the savor and intensity of yesteryear's long distance. An international call requires planning and forethought. First of all, you have to figure out what time it is in another country, and the arithmetic can be daunting.

Patterns of life in other countries are mysterious: we can't easily picture the daily routines, the comings and goings. Reaching a voice oceans away—hearing it live and eager—seems a victory over nearly insuperable odds. Or we might reach a machine: the usual message sounds odd in those foreign syllables, yet it gives a flush of recognition too: Aha! So their lives are like ours; this is what their friends hear all the time.

At last the goal is reached. We speak. And until recently there would come that puzzling little time lag between our speech and the reply, the half-second it took for each voice to stretch its way across the waters. We would speak, but every reply was preceded by a minuscule delay. The faraway person seemed to be hesitating ever so slightly, the sort of hesitation that in ordinary talk means some ambiguous feeling barring the way to a willing response. The conversation had an awkwardness, moving as it did in tiny fits and starts. We felt our words were not being well received, or not being received in the way we intended them. We quickly grasped that this was an electronic, not a personal, lag, but the blight remained. And the feeling was surely mutual: our response never quite satisfying, our timing off.

This small lag embodied the true and broad meaning of distance. However wonderful the magic of electronics, it hadn't closed the gap entirely. Time and space were between us, claiming their reality. You may feel close, they told us, but you are not close. Now even that small gap has been spanned, thanks to more efficient magic. At least I didn't hear it while talking to Italy last week. I missed it. The artisans of Persian carpets, we're told, left a small error in the weave to signify human imperfection. In the same spirit, it was good to be reminded of our separateness and of the uncrossable spaces, not merely between our bodies but between our voices and the words they tenderly, mutually, wistfully bear.

127

"Give Me Your Tired, Your Poor . . ."

As a small child in deepest Brooklyn, post-war, pre-cool Brooklyn, I had many wishes, mostly extravagant and drawn from fantasy, but one of my most fervent was modest and attainable: I wanted permission to cross East New York Avenue by myself. I was allowed to wander around the neighborhood on my own or with friends—parents then were far less anxious and hovering. But East New York Avenue, perpendicular to our narrow street, was forbidden: dauntingly wide, with heavy two-way traffic, a bus route and no traffic light. You had to wait for a break in the swishing parade of cars, as at the Piazza Vittorio Emmanuele in Rome, and then dash across, a leap of faith. When I went back years later I found, as often happens, it was not so wide at all, nothing compared to the broad avenues of Manhattan, never mind Rome.

Finally when I was about eight, I got my wish. My goal was the dim, cramped candy store on the far side of East New York Avenue, with its abundant riches. My father began sending me there to buy him a cigar, and rewarded me with its gold paper ring.

But the privilege carried with it the unlooked-for task of going to Mr. Blustein's grocery store for my mother, next door to the candy store and, like it, the size of a luxurious walk-in closet. I was glad to be judged grown-up enough for this errand—my mother was pregnant, and given her history of miscarriages was advised to stay in bed as much as possible—but I also dreaded it. I was intimidated by Mr. Blustein, the grocer, who sat on a high stool behind a counter surrounded by boxes and cans.

He was squat, barrel-chested, with a jowly, bristly moon face, a grayish complexion, pebbly inscrutable eyes, a bulbous nose and an unlit yet smelly olive-green cigar clamped between his teeth. (My father smoked smelly cigars too, but he never kept them protruding from his mouth once they were dead.) Mr. Blustein's scrunched-up face gathered in folds that seemed to lean toward the cigar. He never smiled and rarely spoke, not even to greet customers. He gave a nod of acknowledgment, more like an upside-down nod, a slight upward tilt of the chin. In response to greetings he would grunt.

Neither my mother nor the other neighborhood women were afraid of Mr. Blustein. If I had told my mother that he scared me, that he was like the ogres in my fairy-tale books, she surely would have laughed. "Mr. Blustein?" I can hear her low, soothing voice. "What could he possibly do to you?" I couldn't explain. He was just so different. The ugliness. The silence. The sense that he was already angry, though I had done nothing wrong yet—not dropped a fruit or knocked over a box. It was his extreme otherness. I was feeling Henry James's reflexive dismay—disgust, really—when he observed the Jewish immigrants on the Lower East Side over a century ago (some of them perhaps my distant relatives), with their overflowing pushcarts, their cluttered syllables, their perceived lack of civilized manners or educated awareness.

Mr. Blustein was an immigrant too, a few steps above the pushcart vendors. An East European Jew, I found out later when I asked my mother why he was so grumpy. He had been through the war, she said, and lost his family. I couldn't imagine Mr. Blustein having children. Ogres didn't have children. In any event, I was a few years older then and knew vaguely

129

that there had been a war. Whispered survivor stories seeped into overheard grown-up conversations: hiding out in cellars or escaping through forests, or simply enduring. But if my mother knew anything of Mr. Blustein's history, she didn't say. My parents almost never spoke of the war in my presence. I learned about it later, as an adolescent, from André Schwartz-Bart's novel, *The Last of the Just*.

Mostly my mother shrugged at my questions. Who knows why people are the way they are? she said. He's probably had a hard time, and he must barely scrape by with that store.

Four or five customers made a crowd. The neighborhood women were loyal to Mr. Blustein despite his sour demeanor. They appreciated his convenient location and his uncanny ability to stock almost everything they needed in that small space, and maybe they were sympathetic. There was no larger store or supermarket nearby; when a supermarket did open a block away, after I'd gone off to college, it probably put him out of business, despite any lingering sympathy. The women waited patiently, not forming a line—that would have been impossible—but in a cluster, remembering the order in which they'd arrived, chatting and gossiping, comparing the qualities of the fruit.

Most of the groceries, the canned or boxed goods, were jammed on shelves behind him; you had to ask Mr. Blustein for whatever you wanted. He rarely moved from his high perch, so that I never saw anything of him below the barrel chest; it was as if he were glued to the stool he sat on. He reached for items by wielding a long pole with pincers on the end. I was enthralled by that pole, which he maneuvered like an implement in some arcane sport, and I would have loved to try it but wouldn't dream of asking. It was like an extension of his fist. He knew his stock so well that, barely turning around, he stretched his arm behind him, the pole attached, and captured the item: Kellogg's cornflakes, Rice Krispies, Bon Ami scouring powder, cans of Del Monte Fruit Cocktail, which my mother often served for dessert, dice-sized cubes of pear and peach in sweet heavy syrup.

Opposite the counter where he presided were wooden crates of fruit, McIntosh apples, Bartlett pears, bananas, huge navel oranges whose skin was all bumps like a severe case of acne. These we would pick out ourselves and bring to the counter to be weighed in the balance scale to Mr. Blustein's left.

I feared setting off his temper—a roaring Fe-Fi-Fo-Fum if I did something wrong, sent the pimpled oranges skittering along the floor or fumbled in reading my list. I was afraid of loud anger because my father lost his temper and shouted all the time, but I knew what provoked him and could avoid it or run upstairs to my room and close the door. Mr. Blustein was an enigma; I had no clue how to protect myself.

Maybe to demystify him, I tried to imagine a story for him, but instead of his troubled past, I preferred to imagine a future. Maybe he'd be shot in his store by teenagers come to rob. He resists. Maybe he kept a gun hidden under the counter, but his ponderous movements were too slow to get it out in time. That he was capable of shooting the thieves, I could well imagine. Angry enough but not agile enough.

What a cruel story. I might have had him act heroically, or at least press an alarm button under the counter to scare the thieves off. It wasn't even an original story but something I'd overheard my parents discussing about an acquaintance who owned a liquor store. Its irony was painfully cheap: surviving the war only to be murdered after passing through our "golden door." In those post-war days every New York City school child had memorized Emma Lazarus's now supersed-

ed poem, "The New Colossus," engraved on a plaque in the
Statue of Liberty, welcoming the "huddled masses yearning
to breathe free."

But with my taste for drama, it wouldn't do to have him
die quietly in his bed, wherever that might be. Maybe he never closed the store, just slept on the stool. I simply wanted to
get rid of him and what he represented, or rather what our
encounters meant about both of us. I resented his invading
my narrow little world with his difference, his pain.

His image remains with me all these years later, floating
uncomfortably in my memory like a lash in the eye. Or rather
a floater, one of those blurry spots that now and then blocks
your vision briefly. I feel ill at ease about my empty encounters with Mr. Blustein. Not that anything in particular was
required of me; nothing more than reading off the groceries
on my mother's list and paying for them. I never spoke to
him aside from that, except for a murmured thank-you, and
that is what makes me blink.

When his chin tilted in my direction indicating my turn
had come, I read off my mother's list timidly, one item at a
time which he plucked grudgingly, or so it seemed, from the
shelves. Sometimes my mother had special requirements,
such as Carolina rice, no other brand, or Tide and not Dreft,
which he'd given me the last time. I was reluctant to try his
patience with her specifications, although when my mother
was with me, she had no such hesitations. She was not just
unafraid, she was even friendly, or as friendly as anyone can
be who expects no response. He provided all she asked for,
without fuss. They might even exchange some words—I
can't recall about what—although Mr. Blustein never went
so far as to remove the cigar from between his teeth.

There was one skill of Mr. Blustein's that impressed me.
Before packing each customer's groceries in a brown paper

bag, he would remove the stubby pencil from behind his hairy left ear, list the cost of each item on the bag and then add up the column at lightning speed, muttering under his breath and moving the pencil downward from one number to the next as if he were drawing a vertical line. He had no cash register; the annotated bag was the receipt. I couldn't help admiring this routine. Not only because Mr. Blustein knew the cost of every item by heart—he never had to consult labels on cans or boxes—but because he could add so supernaturally fast. I still had trouble carrying numbers from the tens to the ones column. At home my mother checked the list on the bag as she took out the items, and she checked his addition too, but never found an error.

Mr. Blustein's arithmetic prowess was doubly uncanny, for it was exactly the way my father, an accountant (many steps up from the pushcarts), added figures in his big ledger spread out on the dining room table. He could go down a long list of figures, three or four digits each, moving his clean, long and sharpened pencil, so different from Mr. Blustein's blunt stubby one, swiftly down the page, also muttering to himself, and finally writing the total at the bottom. I had believed my father possessed a rare skill. It was disconcerting to see that Mr. Blustein could do it too, even though his lists were shorter and written on a humble brown paper bag rather than dignified ledger paper.

My father was an immigrant too, though you would never know it. Aside from the cigars and the superhuman arithmetic, he was nothing like the grocer, and he spoke volubly, in perfect English. I never connected him with the "wretched refuse" whom the Statue of Liberty, in Emma Lazarus's words, was inviting to our "sea-washed gates." But I knew he had been born elsewhere, and I thought maybe that facility for adding columns of figures was something brought over from the Old World, inaccessible to the native born, the way Chinese merchants could use an abacus—this I'd once seen on a family excursion to Chinatown.

Naturally the older I got, the less frightened I was. He was simply the old familiar grocer, no longer a gruesome figure from a fairy tale. I hardly regarded him as a person at all. He was a function. But at some point it occurred to me that although Mr. Blustein and I had known—or rather seen—each other for so long, we had barely exchanged two words besides my reading off the items on my mother's list. And it struck me that this was not the way things should be between people who saw each other once or twice a week for years. I was friendly enough with other shopkeepers—my mother needed my help even more when she became busy with my little brother—but I rarely spoke first. If the shopkeepers spoke to me, asking after my family or making some joke, I could respond in kind. There were even a few stores I liked going to because the owners teased me or complimented me. But I could not initiate anything. I could only wait to be engaged.

Maybe I was a fairy-tale character just as Mr. Blustein had once been, a haughty ice queen or, better still, a princess unable to speak, like some princesses in fairy tales cannot weep or laugh and have to be cured by peeling onions or being shown ridiculous antics. Even today, if I happened to meet Mr. Blustein on the street (impossible; he is surely dead, I hope not by violence), I might not be capable of more than nodding, although I know now that despite his dead cigar and silence and stubbly cheeks, more unites us than separates us, and surface details are no more than a thin skin over a common nature and destiny. I have educated myself out of my fear of difference. I still believe in the forgotten dream of that forgotten poem. I might stop and say hello, but what would I say next?

Floaters in the eye usually go away. But that store and that grocer do not go away, nor does the child I was, blinkered by the willful limits of the provinces, a child for whom the tangible was less real than a story. I have enlightened her, but she trails me like a shadow that even the light of understanding can't erase, too close for comfort.

Time Off to Translate

Strenuous. Grim. Resolute. Blithe. Alluring. Cringe. Recoil. Admonish. The words come from a long list scrawled in my handwriting, four or five at a time in different colored pens, on the blank front pages of an Italian book: *Smoke Over Birkenau*, by Liana Millu. The author, a writer and journalist born in Genoa, spent four months of 1944 imprisoned in Birkenau, the women's part of Auschwitz. When she went home to Italy after the war—one of 57 people to return out of her transport of 672—she wrote her memoir of daily life in the women's camp, in the form of six stories which Primo Levi praised in a 1947 review as "human dilemmas in an inhuman world."

After the first edition in 1947, *Smoke Over Birkenau* went out of print until 1957, when it was reissued, half-heartedly, it seems, by the prominent Italian publisher Mondadori and went the usual way of unpublicized books. In 1979, the author recounts in a letter, she felt something had to be done. "I have no family. I am alone. I realized I couldn't neglect the future of my book." With the help of a friend, Daniel Vogelmann, proprietor of a small publishing firm in Florence called La Giuntina, she brought out two editions. In 1986 La Giuntina published a very successful fifth edition, and a sixth in 1991. Since then the book has been translated into German, French and English.

I spent most of 1990 working on an English translation of *Smoke Over Birkenau*. When I recently opened the Italian edition I worked from, I found the list of words scrawled in the front, in my handwriting. Not long ago, I must have known how they got there and why, but now they were a mystery. Insouciant. Astounded. Hordes. Routine. Perfunctory. Fervent. Vitality. Interminable.

I did the translation in a kind of dream, or nightmare, mentally living four or five hours a day in the extermination camp I conjured up from words on the page, first the Italian, and then my own English words, which made the camp seem closer and more vivid, seen directly rather than through a screen. I didn't think much about why I was doing it. First, why was I doing a translation at all, something bound to be strenuous and difficult, especially as my knowledge of Italian was not as thorough as it should be? Even more, why had I chosen a book that would plunge me into so grim a setting— for more months, as it turned out, than the actual author spent in the actual camp? Only lately have I begun to think about how the work intersected with my life and with my own work, which was writing fiction.

In the fall of 1988, I had finished a novel, and for the next six months, I didn't know what to do with myself. The novel was out of my hands, moving through the various stages of getting printed and bound, for which I was no longer necessary. I tried starting another one but couldn't find any more words. It was as if, in that novel, I had used up all the words I knew, although it was quite short, as novels go. I wrote an unsuccessful story. I was asked to do a few essays and reviews; as always, when writing on demand, I felt I was resolutely completing term papers. I had always wanted to write a musical comedy, so I did the lyrics for several songs, which I still keep in a folder and hope to return to someday; they were funny songs, but I couldn't think of a plot in which they might be set.

I wasn't teaching; there was no place I had to go each day. I would not be missed anywhere since no one expected me. In the morning I would sit down at my desk as a writer should, but that was as far as I got, sitting there and maybe writing a few more blithe verses for my songs. It got so that I would cringe when I awoke and opened my eyes to the light, knowing that yet again I'd have to confront my desk. There were times my body actually recoiled from the desk, and no matter how I admonished myself, I could not produce any useful words.

It was then that I got the notion of translating. I had done some translation years ago and recalled it as serene, absorbing work, wonderful work. It had all the alluring intricacies of writing, the playing with words and phrases and rhythms, except you didn't have to make anything up. That was the best part. You felt you were writing and in a way you were, but the part of the mind that made things up could rest, and obviously that was what my imagination needed. Of course writing—real writing—is also translation, that is, transferring something into one's native tongue, except the language from which one is translating isn't a verbal, audible language.

An astute friend once told me that when you need any of the basics of life—a job, an apartment, or a mate—the first thing to do is tell everyone you encounter that you're looking. I did that. I told everyone who crossed my path that I wanted to translate something from Italian. And sure enough, an Italian friend, a professor of American literature at the University of Florence, soon wrote to say that, at his urging, the Jewish Publication Society had acquired *Smoke Over Birkenau* but had not yet settled on a translator.

I was sent a copy of the book—I remember it was in July 1989—and I read it while on vacation at the beach. It was a strange routine indeed, passing the days in the insouciant ambience of the beach and the evenings reading of the atrocities of the Nazi extermination camps. I found the book enthralling. More important, it was a tangible thing I could do; as I held it in my hands, I felt its shape and bulk could release me from the limbo where I was adrift.

I developed a yen to do it, coupled with apprehension. The language was simple and direct, but I knew how inadequate my Italian was. I would have to look up so many words, even words I was pretty sure of, to be absolutely sure. On the other hand, I had an affinity for the language and its rhythms. I understood the inner shapes of the sentences, their movements and their routes. I almost felt as if Italian were my native tongue, except that I lacked the vocabulary. I had its forms in my head, in the Chomskyesque sense, but not the words. I also had a feeling for how the book should sound in English.

There was still another reason. The subject—the Nazi death camps—was something I thought about a lot, as do many writers, perhaps all thinking people. But it would probably not find a path into my writing except in the most oblique way, since it existed in my life only in an oblique way. Even if I knew what to say, even if I had the skill and imagination, I would still hesitate. I would worry about my ignorance, my possible arrogance in attempting it. The translation would be a way of writing about the camps without actually writing, just as I had not actually lived in them. It would be taking part in some way, doing a small service. It would also be an escape from the need or the desire to write about the subject, just as my having been born when and where I was, was an escape from the reality.

*　　*　　*

Haggard. Cantankerous. Imploring. Dreary. Plucky. Banter. Superb. Vivacious. Snarling. Prattled.

There ensued a lengthy period of correspondence and cantankerous negotiations with the publisher, again a period longer than the time Liana Millu spent in Birkenau. The endless delays were galling, especially as the project was a modest book of one hundred sixty pages, involving a sum of money in the middling four figures.

Toward the end of July, I wrote a letter from the beach saying I'd be interested in doing the book. A few months later, in early fall, I was invited to submit a sample translation of five pages, any five pages I wished. I chose a passage in which a prisoner sneaks out to the camp's black market in the evening to trade a bit of bread for a carrot or piece of onion she could smuggle to her thirteen-year-old son, whom she has discovered, scrawny and haggard, working in the garbage detail in nearby Auschwitz. It was a passage that made the despicable outrage of the camps quite clear, as the imploring mother bargains with fellow prisoners over miserable scraps of food.

It took me two weeks to get the five pages in good shape. If five pages took two weeks, I figured that one hundred sixty pages would take about thirty-two weeks, or eight months.

Early in December, with winter coming on, the beach a distant memory, I received a written offer to do the book. I set myself a goal of five pages a day in very rough form—a literal, not yet literary, translation. As anticipated, I had to look up many words. I had a fat, excellent Italian-English dictionary, and I became so intimate with this dictionary that I could turn automatically to the correct page for the first letter of the word I sought, and soon to the correct page for the first two or three letters of the word. This is no mean feat with a dictionary, particularly with one so thick. (Had I been working on the book ten years later, of course I would have used an online Italian-English dictionary and saved time, yet in retrospect I'm glad I got to know my fat dictionary so well.)

But help was not always to be found in the dictionary—for instance in the story of Bruna, the prisoner who one day spies her half-dead son in neighboring Auschwitz. The narrator, Liana, wonders how she can help Bruna smuggle food to the boy to keep him alive, as well as to make his coming birthday a bit less dreary. She recalls how on her own recent birthday in the camp, a friend with an unquenchable sense of style presented her with "a small slice of salted bread and a tiny bit of margarine," procured by saving up crusts and trading them on the camp's black market. This plucky friend, elegant and freckle-faced, she calls "*la mia amica fiumana.*"

Fiumana, that adjective describing the friend, was a puzzler. It obviously derived from *fiume*, river, and indeed there it was in the dictionary, right after *fiume,* in the *f*s, to which my trained finger turned unerringly. But it was listed as a noun meaning "broad stream" or "large stream"; another meaning was "flood." Figuratively, "*fiumana*" could also mean a crowd or stream of people, as in "a stream of people came out of the theater." "My streaming friend"? No, that wouldn't do.

I spent some time pondering this freckled, stylish *amica fiumana*. She must have had a generous, vivacious nature, since in such straitened circumstances she'd managed to give the narrator that gift of bread and margarine. "My generous friend"? No, the author would simply have called her *generosa*. There was more to it. "My bountiful friend"? I was leaning toward "my exuberant friend," trying to keep the river-like, overflowing sense contained in the word. But I wasn't satisfied. I happened to mention my problem on the phone to the

Italian professor who had gotten me involved in the project to begin with. "*Fiumana?*" he repeated, amused. "From Fiume."

Fiume is a Northern Italian city and *fiumana* was a simple adjective of location like *romana* (Roman) or *fiorentina* (Florentine). What threw me off was that, in Italian, adjectives derived from proper nouns are not capitalized. Of course, I knew this elementary fact but, because of my geographical ignorance, never thought to apply it to the situation at hand. Meanwhile, being a novelist, I had developed a whole identity for this friend who exists in a mere four lines—bountiful, exuberant, with long flowing hair and moist, brimming eyes and an undulating way of moving. A common practice of fiction writers is: when you don't know something, make it up. But it clearly wasn't going to be the proper strategy for a translator.

In the end, the narrator decides to emulate her bountiful friend from Fiume and persuades the other women in the barrack to put aside a morsel of bread each day for a week. By this means they amass enough bread to trade on the black market for a clove of garlic for the boy's birthday; his mother is overcome with gratitude.

For all I knew, people from Fiume might be noted for their generosity and exuberance, their lush features and fluid grace, the way, for example, people from New York are noted (mistakenly) for their brusque manners and haste and snarling speech. At any rate, I realized that to avoid similar errors, I needed help. A translation therapist, so to speak. For the last year or so there had been ads on the New York City buses for psychological services. "Let's face it," the ads said. "Emotional problems don't go away by themselves." Well, neither do translation problems. I needed someone to elucidate turns of phrase, offhand jokes and references that are clear only to native speakers or insiders. I had lived in Italy for a year, long ago, but that wasn't enough.

I thought immediately of Francesco, a language teacher I had lately made friends with. Francesco was thirty-two years old and a polyglot. True, he was not a native speaker of Italian—he was from the Bronx—but he had grown up speaking it with his Italian father, as well as speaking Spanish with his mother, who was Dominican. Along the way, at Cardinal Spelman High School in the Bronx and later at Cornell, he had picked up Latin, French and Portuguese. When it came to matters linguistic, Francesco was the ultimate authority. During his first few years out of college, he had worked for a bank, where he was a most valuable employee since he could be sent anywhere in the world: if he didn't already speak the language, he'd pick it up in a few minutes.

It was plain to see that Francesco was not born to bank. He was slender and sprite-like, full of vitality, with quick, lithe movements—rather like the friend from Fiume. He had darkish skin, straight coal-black hair and a gap between his teeth; he had huge dark soulful eyes, and he was warm and ebullient, full of laughter and banter. He read religion and philosophy and was a fervent believer who went to church regularly—a Protestant church, not the church of his parents. He had also studied history and knew the dates and names of everything that had ever happened in Western Europe and perhaps elsewhere. After a few years in a business suit, he'd quit the bank and begun giving language lessons; that way he could wear jeans and his superb and colorful silk shirts.

I imagined bringing the translation to him for help: we could sit in the tiny living room of his fifth-floor walk-up, or else climb the spiral staircase to the room with the birds: he kept two finches in a cage, and if they made too much noise when he had friends or students over, he would spread a towel over the cage to make them think it was night, and the gullible creatures would immediately shut up. Or we might go out on the roof terrace, which he'd decorated with thriving plants and colored banners—red, purple, green, pink, blue and yellow—and look out over the city as I told him my translation problems and he listened with sympathetic nods.

But Francesco said regretfully that he was too busy with students and suggested someone else, a young Italian woman across town. Her name sounded familiar. I remembered I had known a couple by that name when I lived in Rome in the 1960s. There might be no connection at all, but then again it was an unusual name. I went to her apartment and asked her if her parents' names were Dora and Ruggiero. Yes, they were. "I knew your parents in Rome," I said in astonishment. "We were friends. I knew your mother even before that, back in Philadelphia. In fact, I think I even babysat for you once or twice. Were you a year or two old in 1964?" "Yes," she said, "that must have been me."

She was pleasant enough, but she didn't seem astounded at the coincidence as I was, or even terribly interested. Her manner was perfunctory, as I prattled on about how I'd stayed at her parents' beach house in Fregene and looked after her and her sister as a favor—I was hardly more than a girl myself then. I grasped that while it was for me indeed an astounding coincidence to be referred to the daughter—living unaccountably in New York—of friends I'd known almost thirty years ago in Rome, for her it was simply running into an old friend of her parents, ho-hum.

Insipid. Puny. Taunt. Rejoinder. Seethed. Rancid. Drab. Halting. Surly.

I had met the young translation therapist's American mother, Dora, shortly after I graduated from college: she was the personnel director who interviewed me for a typing job at the American Friends Service Committee in Philadelphia. I had recently married and was to be the breadwinner while my husband went to graduate school.

Typing for a Quaker social service agency was not my first choice. Since I'd been an English major in college, I had initially looked in the field of publishing, specifically Curtis Publishing Company, whose headquarters were in Philadelphia and which published the *Saturday Evening Post* and other popular magazines of the day. The interviewer at Curtis—I remember her still, a bony woman in a narrow, insipid little dress with a cap of dark hair that clung to her puny head—raised her eyes from my résumé and said, as if it were a taunt, "I see you are married." In those days such information was included on résumés. "Yes," I acknowledged. "If you're married," she countered, "you might get pregnant." That was definitely a rebuke.

I could hardly dispute the bare statement. "But I don't plan to get pregnant for a long time," I said. "'The best laid plans of mice and men go oft astray,'" was her rejoinder.

Fresh from college and steeped in English literature, I might have told her that the line she misquoted was actually "The best-laid schemes o' mice an' Men, Gang aft a-gley." But I didn't have the presence of mind. I seethed with outrage. In those days we didn't know that what she was doing was a form of discrimination, of sexism, as well as intimidation. Or was it? Is injustice abstract? Does it exist before it is officially recognized as such? Well, that is a metaphysical question, like the tree falling in the forest. In any case I felt very badly used, but at the time there wasn't anything I could do about my rejection. It's possible that enough of those encounters might make a young woman go out and get pregnant in a fit of spite, to fulfill the prophecy. I left the Curtis building with the rancid taste of injustice on my tongue.

I wasn't too successful at hunting up jobs. Another I applied for was in a laboratory, removing the legs from fruit flies, the kind you swat in the kitchen. The man who interviewed me was a drab person with halting speech. "You know about fruit flies?" he mumbled. "*Drosophila melanogaster*." As a matter of fact, I did know, even though I was an English major. I remembered from high school biology that because of certain physical characteristics, and perhaps also because of their ubiquity, fruit flies were commonly used for experiments in genetics. Not only had Mendelian genetics been one of the few topics in biology that interested me, but I liked the fruit flies' Latin name: *Drosophila melanogaster*. Perhaps they are still used, though with the enormous advances in genetics and the Genome Project, they have probably been superseded.

Despite a certain repugnance, I was considering taking the fruit fly job with the mumbling scientist, when I was offered the typing job at the American Friends Service Committee by Dora, future mother of the translation therapist. Typing was not what I'd had in mind all those years I pored over English literature, but it seemed preferable to fruit flies. I had tried to rationalize the fruit fly job by telling myself I'd be contributing to genetic research, and now I tried to rationalize the typing job by telling myself I'd be contributing to peace in the world, for the Quakers who ran the AFSC were doing a variety of good works in poor countries. But I think what clinched it was the vision of myself interminably plucking the legs from fruit flies—after all, who knew how long it might take my husband to finish his graduate studies?

At the AFSC, Dora was kind to me. She saw to it that after six months as a typist I was promoted upstairs to the

Foreign Service section as a secretarial assistant. I worked for a man who administered a work camp program in Europe: we processed the applications of hordes of American college students who hoped to spend the summer living in Spartan conditions while digging wells or building schools or libraries in poor European towns, some still feeling the devastation of the war. I was barely older than the students going to the camps, and my boss—a gentle, innocent Quaker I thought of as elderly but who was probably about fifty-five—occasionally asked if I wouldn't want to try a work camp myself.

I said no, I didn't care to sleep in a sleeping bag and eat cheap starchy food cooked communally in enormous pots and dig ditches for six weeks. I was an English major through and through, and innocent as he was, he soon came to grasp this. "Oh, but a human being can stand anything for six weeks," he would tease. "I'm not so sure," I retorted.

It was 1960. Little by little over the past decade, details about the extermination camps had begun seeping into the public consciousness. When he said, "A human being can stand anything for six weeks," I immediately thought of Auschwitz and Dachau. I couldn't foresee that, in later life, once I had escaped being a typist and become a writer, I would learn Italian and one day translate a book about Auschwitz. But I would sometimes imagine myself imprisoned there, in those hellish conditions, and did not think I'd be among the ones who endured. I was too hot-tempered and impatient—I would anger a surly guard, who would shoot me. Now I am no longer so hot-tempered, and when I imagine myself there, I think I might have the patience but not the physical stamina to endure. They'd take one look at me and, with a perfunctory wave of the hand, send me off to the bad side.

In one of the six stories in *Smoke Over Birkenau*, which I was to translate longer than I typed for the AFSC, an eighteen-year-old Dutch prisoner named Lotti understands quite well that some human beings can't bear certain conditions. Watching her sister sicken and wither in the camp, Lotti volunteers to work in the Nazi brothel. When her dying sister disowns her in shame, Lotti justifies her choice in an ardent speech about her passion to stay alive by any means. She quotes from the Book of Job: "'As the cloud is consumed and vanisheth away, so he that goeth down to the grave shall come up no more. He shall return no more to his house.' 'Well,'" Lotti protests, "'I refused to be consumed and vanish like a cloud. I wanted to return to my house. I'm eighteen years old—I don't want to die. I know, no one wants to die, you'll tell me. But maybe I don't want to more than the others. Maybe that's the difference.'"

I was not only moved but alarmed when I came across this passage. It was hard enough to translate a contemporary Italian author. Must I tackle the Bible as well? What grave misgivings I suffered, until it dawned on me that the Bible had already been translated into English. All I had to do was locate the passage and copy it.

The act of copying felt sneaky. Fiction writers store many beloved snatches from other writers in their heads, often for so long that we feel we've written them ourselves. We learn to be wary about what we appropriate. Even though it was perfectly legitimate in this case, I lifted from the Book of Job with unease.

Meanwhile, when my Quaker boss teased me, back in 1960, saying, "A human being can stand anything for six weeks," I replied, "I'm not so sure." He looked perplexed; he really thought a human being could stand anything for six weeks—a tribute to the innocence of his imagination—and I did not enlighten him. He was a mild man; I wasn't sure he could stand my fantasies about the camps for even a few minutes.

I worked listlessly at the AFSC for two years and, because of the innocence I perceived there, was probably the only employee who never attended the optional silent meeting held every morning before work. I also liked to sleep late. Toward the end of my tenure, I did finally attend a few silent meetings at Pendle Hill, a Quaker retreat outside of Philadelphia, where our work campers came for a week of orientation and where I was permitted to use some of my college education in teaching rudimentary French classes. The silent meetings were fine, a curiosity, and I regretted my two-year intransigence, but I was disturbed by an evening talk given by one of the high-ranking AFSC executives. (As a Quaker group, the AFSC wasn't supposed to have ranks but it did nonetheless, and everyone tacitly understood and observed them, for example in the company lunchroom, where one was invited to sit anywhere but the executives always sat at certain tables and the secretaries at others.)

The talk was about pacifism. It was a very nice talk—Quakers and pacifism can be appealing—but during the question and answer period one of the students asked, as people invariably do, about Hitler. What would you do about Hitler? "Hate the deed and not the doer," the high-ranking executive replied in his rasping voice. He said it as if he had been asked that question many times and was tired of it, even rankled—Why do they keep harping on that? I imagined him thinking—and had his answer prepared to deliver by rote. As if on cue, I walked out and strolled through the pleasant suburban grounds in the warm evening.

After I left my secretarial assistant's job at the AFSC, I went to graduate school. What else, if typing and fruit flies were my only career options? I needed two languages for a master's degree and decided to study Italian on my own. Languages had always come easily to me, and all I needed was enough to pass a reading comprehension exam. It was a happy choice, for two years later I found myself living in Rome. There I looked up Dora, who had also left the AFSC, married a Roman, moved to Italy and had two babies, whom I would take care of a few times in gratitude for her invitations to the beach house in Fregene, and one of whom, decades later, would become my translation therapist.

I couldn't stop thinking about the convoluted trail of coincidence leading me back to Dora and her Italian daughter. It nagged at me with mounting intensity, the way a story idea nags. It wasn't the coincidence as such that I found so compelling, after my initial surprise, as the discrepancy between my reaction to it and that of the translation therapist. It was interesting, in the Jamesian sense of the word, that the same situation could be so striking to one party involved, evoking whole chunks of the past, and so negligible to the other. And yet in this situation the discrepancy was natural and understandable.

Misgivings. Listless. Rasping. Harping. Wary. Capitulate. Cue. Immersed. Mounting.

As I got deeper into the translation and could navigate in the author's idiom, the English version emerged and, with it, the sensation that I myself was writing the book. I had familiar urges to cut, to revise, to sharpen and expand dialogue, move paragraphs around and make verbal links. I would see an opportunity for a metaphor or an analogy, or an opening where characters from earlier stories might reappear speaking new words. I had to keep myself from capitulating to such urges. The text came to seem a constraint. What felt most peculiar was not the urge to cut but the opposite urge to expand. Maybe just another phrase or so here . . . I'd think, and on the verge of inventing something, would suddenly remember I wasn't the writer. I wasn't allowed to invent. Moreover, the book wasn't really fiction, or fiction only in the loosest sense; it was a memoir, no doubt adorned and enhanced, but the events had really happened. Besides being only the translator, I couldn't expand because I didn't know any more than what was given on the page. I hadn't been there. It wasn't my memoir.

While I was immersed in the translation, I went to the MacDowell Colony in New Hampshire. Now, writers go to these colonies to write, not to translate, and even though no one checks your daily output, you do feel an obligation at least to try to write. I even wanted to write. It was almost spring, and I finally had words; I had a new novel in mind. But I had contracted to do the Birkenau book, and so I established a routine. I would spend the mornings on my allotted five pages of the translation, which was coming to feel interminable—the roll calls, the brutal labor, the hard crusts of bread and watery soup, the beatings, the selections, the smoke rising from the crematoria—and the afternoons on my novel.

But something happened to disrupt my well-laid plans. They went astray, as the prim interviewer at Curtis Publishing might say. A part of my mind that was not routinized stealthily came up with a story parallel to my situation with Dora's daughter, the translation therapist. What other pair of people might have similarly polar reactions to a chance connection? I imagined a man, a diffident, unformed young man, going to Italy, having a brief unforgettable love affair, returning home to resume his humdrum life, and years later meeting a young Italian woman who he realizes is his daughter. Francesca would be her name. He doesn't tell her the whole truth, only that he knew her parents years ago in Rome. To him, the coincidence is astounding and impels him to review his entire life. To her, it's nothing much.

Bemused, I began pacing around my chilly MacDowell studio as the story took on vitality. I dropped my routine to write it and called it "Francesca." It turned out, as stories do, to be about many other and more complex things than the discrepancy in two characters' perception of a coincidence. And any of its other strands might be traced back through my life in a meandering quest much like this one.

Stealthy. Bemused. Upbraided. Pacing. Predicament. Gasp. Runt. Deserted.

Beyond its fictional offshoots, the translation generated scores of problems, all of which I had to work out myself. For a translation therapist is like any therapist—she cannot do the difficult thing for you; she can only offer information and a disinterested view, maybe setting the problem in a more auspicious context.

The problems began with the very first sentence. A raw literal translation would be: "There was a bit of consternation that morning because there had been a medical check the night before, and many girls had been sent to the sand block." Those "girls," for openers. The book had been written in 1946, a time when men were men and women were . . . girls. People like the interviewer at Curtis did their damage unchallenged. But no longer. There was no way I could refer to a group of women doing hard labor and facing imminent death, many grieving for the husbands they had left behind and the children torn from them, as girls. Yes, quite a few were in their late teens, but most were in their twenties and thirties, and one major character and several minor ones seemed around fifty. The real girls—children—had been destroyed before they ever reached the camp or at its gates.

I agonized over the word, trying to be true simultaneously to the author's vision, to the idiom of the contemporary reader, and to my own convictions. Generally, when seeking the right word, my principle had been to imagine how the writer would express herself were English her native tongue. But I had no idea how Liana Millu, over seventy now, felt about American feminism or the politics of language; perhaps at her age any woman under thirty or even forty seemed a girl.

I tried it both ways—"women" and "girls"—and in the end took a liberty. Whenever "girls" didn't sit right with me, and by extension with my imagined readers, whenever it felt distracting or alienating, I used "women." I also used "women" when referring to the characters in groups. But I kept Millu's "girl" when the character was a teenager, as in, "two rows away stood a very young, pretty girl with a friendly smile," and in the case of the two sisters, one of whom dies of hunger while the other goes to the well-fed Nazi brothel: not only did "girls" seem all right given their age, but the poignancy of the word heightened the pain of their predicament.

Also in that first sentence, the girls or women "had been sent to the sand block." On receiving my manuscript, the editor wrote and asked, What is this sand block? Well, I replied, it says exactly that, "*block della sabbia*." *Block* was the German word used throughout for the barracks where the women slept. Many prisoners worked in the sand pits, pointlessly hauling truckloads of sand back and forth. I could only assume "the sand block" referred to the barracks housing those women who worked in the pits. I agreed, though, that the phrase was vaguer than Millu's usual style. And in English it had an auditory suggestion of "sandbox," which was very inopportune.

Imagine our surprise when, the book already set in galleys, a letter arrived from Daniel Vogelmann, the Italian publisher. I wonder if I mentioned, he wrote, that in the 1986 edition there were two typos. It wasn't the "*block della sabbia*" at all, but the "*block della scabbia*." "*Scabbia*" (I had to look it up in my fat dictionary) means "scabies." That is, after "the medical check of the night before," many women had been sent to be disinfected for scabies, and thus the confusion in the barracks. Who would have thought it?

A reference to scabies was a fine opening stroke on the author's part, almost lost to something blander and ambiguous. It makes one wonder about all the enduring works of fiction passed down through centuries, painstakingly copied by hand—or maybe not so painstakingly—and what similar misreadings might be serving as the pillars of Western thought.

The other typo was the same perilous, just possible, kind. A young woman in the camp tried to conceal her pregnancy—a forbidden condition in Birkenau—by binding up her stomach with rags to make it look flat. Unwilling to submit to the required abortion, she fervently hopes the war will end in time for her to have her baby at home. She tells the narrator how hard it is to carry the heavy loads assigned to her: "*I sacchi di acqua, i sacchi del pane, i sacchi della paglia*"—sacks of water, sacks of bread, sacks of straw.

Water is not carried in sacks. Yet given the camps' surreal absurdities, the fact that idiotic and impossible tasks were demanded simply to destroy morale, it might just be. I don't recall what I was planning to do about those sacks of water; one mediocre way out might have been to have the character complain about "loads" of water, bread, and straw.

"Not '*sacchi*,'" Vogelmann wrote, but '*secchi*.' Buckets. A single letter made the difference between the absurd and the ordinary. (Had I been a native speaker, I likely would have spotted the error and corrected it automatically.) And yet the notion of carrying water in a sack is less absurd than the actuality of being forced to conceal a pregnancy and haul buckets of water all day for being born into a race scheduled for extermination.

More trouble arose when the narrator and Lili, the "young, very pretty girl with a friendly smile," visit the barrack of an exotic Tunisian prisoner, Madame Louise, the camp's fortune-teller. For a slice of bread or a few leaves of cabbage, the enigmatic Madame Louise will read the tarot cards. She predicts a long journey for Lili, so long that she can't even see the end of it. Lili is overjoyed: she imagines going home to her mother. I managed the intricate laying out of the cards—hearts, spades, the wicked Queen of Spades. But I was stumped when Madame Louise laid out an ominous card she called the "*stella*," or star. It wasn't clubs or diamonds. The dictionary was no help. Even the translation therapist was baffled. I thought of Francesco, my polyglot friend who knew everything.

"Pentagram," he said over the phone, without hesitation. Pentagram. I'd never have gotten it. I would have committed a worse blunder than sacks of water. And I envisioned his fifth-floor walk-up apartment, the crowded living room, the spiral staircase, the birds, the roof terrace with the lush plants and brightly colored streamers, and wished he were helping me, bounding about the room as he liked to do, talking of history and politics and books and movies in his exuberant way, his dark fluid eyes ever attentive.

* * *

Whisked. Piteously. Incorrigible. Reprisals. Gaping. Gross. Furtive. Chide.

Smoke Over Birkenau reflects a polyglot world, dotted with phrases from the various languages spoken in the camp—what we'd call today a multicultural text. In keeping with the author's choice, I left such phrases as they were, now and then giving their meaning unobtrusively in parentheses or a footnote where I feared American readers might be puzzled. For instance, the story about the two Dutch sisters, one dying in the infirmary and the other working in the brothel, is called, "*Scheiss Egal*," a German phrase equivalent in English to "the same old shit."

It was easy enough to explain that title in a note. But when the phrase appeared in the story, used by a middle-aged SS man visiting the brothel, I hit a snag. Liana, the narrator, has just told Lotti, the young prostitute, that her sister is dying. As Lotti weeps, the SS man, hurriedly unbuckling his belt to get down to business, grumbles, "Her sister is sick? Who gives a shit? Always the same old shit!"

"That atrocious, despairing phrase," the narrator comments, "that they would repeat day in and day out, as if to confer on Cambronne's words the dignity of a philosophy."

Who was this Cambronne whose name is dropped so casually, as if every reader ought to know? And what were his words? I tried the encyclopedia. A French general who served under Napoleon. Present at the defeat at Waterloo. So? I called a French friend, who had a good laugh when she heard my question. General Cambronne earned immortality, she told me, by his famous remark at the battle of Waterloo: *Merde*. Since then every French schoolchild has been scolded at one time or another for uttering what is called "*le mot Cambronne.*" I hadn't thought of asking Francesco, and I wonder now if he would have known.

Cambronne became a small but, to me, crucial footnote to the text. Whenever I succeeded in solving some such tiny problem, I felt a great delight, the same delight I knew from my own writing when things suddenly fell into place. An instant later I felt a twinge, resembling guilt, at the bizarre discrepancy of my response. I was so tickled to be able to get it right, so transported by the gifts of language, that I lost sight of the dreadful subject—in this case the German officer's unbuckling his belt to make use of the grieving girl—a scene for which language was only the means, the translation.

The author quoted songs, too, in several languages, for despite their wretchedness, the characters would occasionally sing as they worked, or sing to cheer each other up, or sing during the few hours' rest on Sunday afternoon. One musical woman even sleeps with a German kapo in exchange for a harmonica, along with a few slices of bread. But when the songs were translated into Italian, they needed to be rendered in English, as in the story of Lili, who is nicknamed for the familiar German war song, "Lili Marlene." It was Lili who, according to the tarot cards, would be taking a long journey, so long that Madame Louise couldn't even see the end of it.

The pungent lyrics of "Lili Marlene" became emblematic of the characters' situation. After the Bible episode, I realized right away that these lyrics existed in an English translation. Hunting for them took me to the Library of the Performing Arts at Lincoln Center in New York, where I waited in a cozy armchair while the librarian whisked off behind locked doors to fetch my request. She handed me a mound of tattered old sheet music from the 1940s and I whiled away the afternoon, transported back half a century and enchanted by the songs printed in innocent old typefaces with period illustrations.

The other songs in the text were originally Russian and Dutch, and since it wasn't feasible to visit the Russian and Dutch versions of the Lincoln Center Library of the Performing Arts, I translated them as best I could. This was a treat; I was growing nostalgic for my own work, and almost felt I was back in the lyrics for my nonexistent musical comedy.

Consorting with the kapos wasn't unusual; the women prisoners did it not only for bread, but to snatch a few moments of pleasure in a doomed life, or to have a possible ally during a selection for the gas chambers. Because of their desperation, I needed to know the proper declensions—masculine, feminine, singular and plural—for the Polish word "*kochany*," meaning lover, or more informally, boyfriend or girlfriend. A Polish-English dictionary was no help, so I went to the Slavic languages department at Columbia University, hoping a kind professor might come to my aid. I was so disappointed to find no one in that I moaned piteously to the secretary, a plump blonde woman who seemed a tolerant sort. "All I wanted was the right spelling for a few simple Polish words." "Is that all?" she said. "I'm Polish. What do you need to know?" The experience not only corroborated but extended my astute friend's maxim: Tell everyone you meet what you're looking for, even if it isn't one of the basics such as a job, an apartment, or a mate, but merely the word for mate.

My last foray away from the dictionary was to the YIVO Institute in New York City to find the English terminology for the different work groups in the camps—Commandos, as they were called in Nazi military argot. The YIVO Institute, a center for the study of the Holocaust, was at that time housed in a stately Fifth Avenue mansion with marble walls and a magnificently curving wrought-iron staircase in the lobby. It contained endless shelves of documentation—war reports, statistical breakdowns of prisoners by nationality, age, and sex, as well as by how they died, with photographs. Here, too, I spent an afternoon mesmerized by old books and papers, though not as happily as in the Library of the Performing Arts with the sheet music. I didn't find what I needed and ended up fudging it, but I found something else: a chart showing the Nazis' division of prisoners into categories with distinct identifying marks. A red triangle sewn on the uniform meant political prisoners, a purple triangle meant Jehovah's Witnesses, green was for criminals, pink was for homosexuals, black for "anti-social" types, blue for immigrants, and yellow for Jews, though in this last case an additional triangle was superimposed to form a six-pointed star. A Rainbow Coalition.

I've thought a good deal about the list of words scrawled in my handwriting in the front of the book in different colored pens, signifying that the entries were made at different times. Interminable. Outrage. Stampede. Rancid. And so on. It's true many of the words suit the text and appear in my English version, but others do not. I think they weren't simply suggested by the Italian, but were words I liked and hoped to find an opportunity to use, like an heiress seeking social occasions to display her collection of jewelry. That sounds a trifle frivolous, I know, especially for a translator. How can words come first? What about the truth of a piece of writing, its meaning or content?

Well, a writer's real allegiance is to language, words and their proper placement, without which there is no truth or meaning. The list reminds me that along with the given of Millu's stories, the translation is built out of the English lexicon, the way bricks and mortar make walls to house life.

Shortly after the translation was published, my polyglot friend Francesco died of AIDS at thirty-five years old. He would have worn a pink triangle. When he was sick and I visited him in his fifth-floor walk-up apartment with the caged finches and the plants and colored banners on the roof, I saw lying on a table the copy of the translation which I'd given him. Only he had known the name for the pentagram in the tarot deck, the card Madame Louise said meant a long journey, so long that she couldn't even see the end of it.

Visiting the YIVO Institute, I knew immediately that the information about the colored triangles, the rainbow of prisoners, would become a poem. Sometimes the form of a piece of writing or the images by which it will travel will hit you before anything else. When I wrote it, a few years later, it became another instance of the finite time during which I worked on the translation stretching out and arching, bending as physicists tell us time does when viewed under the aspect of eternity, reaching its tentacles back and forth over my life to encompass it all in a vast and flexible hand.

Detective Briscoe of the NYPD

Caravans of white movie trailers colonizing our streets no longer set me all atwitter. You never see real filming, just guys in jeans carrying cups of take-out coffee. But one morning last year was an exception.

I was ambling down Broadway, around 104th Street, in my pre-noon somnambulistic state, only half-aware of a flurry of movement around me. Suddenly, barely eight feet ahead were two very familiar figures: Detectives Ed Green and Lennie Briscoe (otherwise known as Jesse Martin and the late, great Jerry Orbach), looking larger in life than on screen, heads together, no doubt conferring over the latest body found in the shrubbery in nearby Riverside Park.

I'd walked onto a *Law & Order* set. Of course: I'd watched the show so often and so faithfully that I'd finally crossed the border from life to art.

Lennie caught sight of me. "Out of the way!" he snarled with an impatient wave, exactly as he did on the show when bystanders edged too close to the crime scene. There was no arguing with that deep, petulant croak. I scurried off.

New York is full of sightings, but this was different. It wasn't Jerry Orbach addressing me but the character he'd created and so thoroughly inhabited: Lennie Briscoe, the Jonathan Swift of the NYPD, quintessential tough-skinned, nasty-tongued, brokenhearted New Yorker. ("You think Manhattan's a wasteland? Wait till you see Riker's Island.") Moments later I was firing off emails to my cohort of *L & O* fans—my two daughters, my niece, and my brother. "He spoke to me! He ordered me out of the way!" Within the hour, four suitably impressed responses came back.

Orbach's utterly authentic portrayal of Lennie Briscoe had the power to entrance otherwise sophisticated adults because he was one of us, exponentially enlarged. More than street-smart, a street wizard. He'd seen it all; his face and stance showed it. The watery eyes pleading for a decent night's sleep. The side-of-the-mouth sneer, the weary face etched with pain. Life had roughed him up. Two failed marriages (or, as he put it, "two priors, no convictions"), a struggle with alcoholism ("I've always said drinking alone is underrated"), and the great grief—his daughter killed by a drug-world connection. He didn't talk about that much, but we understood it was what scored his face and made his shoulders slump.

For thirteen years Lennie Briscoe was so vivid and beloved a presence that it was easy to forget the Bronx-born Orbach's distinguished film and musical-comedy career before he took up police work. Just two weeks ago I happened to catch the old film *Dirty Dancing* on TV. Younger, trimmer, with bet-ter posture and hair not yet gray, Orbach plays a self-righteous doctor and father of two naïve teen-aged girls. Enter cognitive dissonance. What was he doing on a Catskills golf course? He belonged on the streets of New York in his aging trench coat, grabbing a hot dog from a stand, bemoaning his marital histo-ry and besotted past, dragging his tired ass all over the city to solve the cases ripped from the headlines.

Lennie dropped in at construction sites, auto repair shops, strip joints, Madison Avenue boutiques, Bronx cab dispatch offices, Chinatown markets. He went from Lower East Side crack houses to university campuses (often my neighbor, Columbia, thinly disguised as "Hudson University"); he visited posh East Side schools and Harlem's basketball courts, Russian Mafia dens in Brighton Beach ("What's Russian for 'you're under arrest'?") and carcass-lined refrigerators in the Meat Packing District. And all in the service of a job that—he never stopped reminding us—paid little and was unappreciated.

In the first three minutes of the show, Lennie's bleary eyes would gaze unwillingly at the corpse—shot, cut, pummeled, poisoned, you name it—with a blend of pity and profound disgust. Then he would utter the wisecrack we all waited for. A student? "She can forget about midterms." A pack of cigarettes in the pocket? "That's one way to kick the habit." To an outlander this might sound insensitive. Sure it is. Lennie can't afford sensitivity—the misery is too unrelenting. Besides, the cracks are funny. Who can resist, living on these streets?

In the tenth season of *L & O*, Lennie promised, "I plan on doing this job in my wheelchair." Yet last spring he retired from the force. How could he? I'd not yet forgiven him (especially as he was slated to appear on another spinoff, *Law & Order: Trial by Jury*) when I learned of Jerry Orbach's death on December 28. The next night, though, he was back on the screen, snarling and smirking. A gift. A stab in the heart. It needed a Lennie-type wisecrack about what dies and what endures.

I live across from hilly Morningside Park. The other day, neighbors looking down from the railing saw a blanket covering a mound, the ground around it stained dark. The police said a homeless man had been knifed in the wee hours. Maybe one of our locals—there was no way to tell. The case never made the headlines. Everyone said the useless words you say in collective sadness. But we were still New Yorkers. "Someone ought to call Lennie," one woman murmured.

A Sort of Hero

The following selection is narrated in the voice of Robert Walser (1878–1956), the great eccentric Swiss writer who left hundreds, if not thousands, of brief essays—whimsical, melancholy, and unique—in addition to several novels. He spent the last years of his life in a mental institution.

My hero was born in a snowstorm; fast and furious fell the downy flakes round his pink young head as he uttered his first piercing shriek, to the delight of his stalwart lady mother, naturally somewhat in disarray from her recent efforts, but nonetheless overjoyed. Into the room dashed his six lively, rosy Alpine brothers and sisters, to be introduced and predict his illustrious future. One of the cleverer sisters, taking a first excited glance at the hushed infant, his eyes already bemused by the multiple wonders displayed before them, pronounced him "not of coarse enough cut for this life." As for the young fellow, he pondered already, as he was to continue to ponder: "What made life so? Is it going to stay as it is, or change? Why am I asking this? Why do so many questions come to me, softly, one after the other?"

Was there really a snowstorm, you may reasonably pause to ask, even at this infantile stage of our chronicle, as it was the month of April? Since I make up the story as it proceeds, I would have it an unseasonable snowstorm, if you please. If I may beg your indulgence, for the simple reason, if I am not sweeping too far ahead of my story, like a train sweeping past the desperate passengers running tardily alongside, hanging on to their hats, that he was to meet his death in the snow. How comforting, isn't it, to have stories come full circle, as in the old high days of narrative? Perhaps if I draw a rounded circle instead of letting my tale evaporate like a little cloud, some lordly publisher will deign to print this frivolous enterprise and not float it fleetly back to me like a paper airplane on billows of wind.

Walser was the name of this fine hero of mine, and hero he was, for he was destined to follow the noble profession of servant, that is to say, writer. What is more noble than the servant who humbles his will and learns to present all things with deftness and agility, whether his task is to carry a whiskey and soda on a silver salver to his most dignified and wealthy employer, or to deposit bushels of harvested words in the ample lap of Poetry's exacting mistress? Indeed, our hero was schooled in humility from his earliest years when his mother loved him, let us say, adequately, but perhaps not quite to the ultimate degree.

On a smiling summer's day, a morning of gay birdsong and beckoning leaves, he set forth through the forests of his native land to seek his fortune. This he did not find so very quickly, it seems, as happens to the best of lads. A handsome, clever youth was he, though perhaps a trifle eccentric or careless in his dress: he did not always replace his buttons as promptly as might be desired or iron his shirts and trousers; he could be seen in the village with an odd assortment of hats of the most distressing colors—orange, blue, grassy green, not at all hatlike.

And yet he cut an amiable figure as he ambled through the streets on his everlasting promenades, observing each flower turn its luscious, colorful, tearful face to the sun, each pious shopkeeper open his doors to the gracious public, while the town stretched its limbs and blinked awake, preparing to endure yet another promising day.

He was unfailingly courteous to all he approached. He gazed with humility and appreciation at the bosoms and bustles of the ladies strolling by on their ladylike errands, some of whom gave back a puzzled glance. He would pause to stroke a peripatetic canine, that is to say, a stray dog, in the spirit of soulful camaraderie. So what if, as he reported, "Nothing ever happened! To be bored and to ponder how I can possibly break the boredom—that is what my real occupation is." Walking, he listened to the murmur of the soul, for "one listens to the murmur of the soul only because of boredom."

Bored or not, he was industrious; we cannot, no, we certainly must not hint that he was unindustrious or—can it even be whispered?—lacking in ambition. He tried his untried hand at a variety of trades; he trod the boards of the stage for a time, he was amanuensis to an inventor, and on occasion settled briefly into the time-honored profession of clerk.

Ah, to be a clerk in a bank, ladies and gentlemen, indulgent readers: Imagine, for a moment, our gifted young hero admitted into the halls of commerce, to shiver to the rustle of bills and the clink of coins, poised at the magnificent center of the modern universe. To be a clerk is to perch on a high stool, pen in hand, and set columns of splendid numbers dancing elegantly across the luxuriant pages of a ledger, to the unheard music, like the music of the spheres, of investment and profits. To be a clerk is to wake in the morning in a small, bare room, don one's dark clerkly garb, fervently swallow one's tea and roll, wave a friendly goodbye to one's tight-lipped landlady wrecked with loneliness, and set out briskly through the morning streets with a missionful purpose . . .

and energy! To be a clerk is to know life, to bow one's head to the inevitable, to the desk. Why, to be a clerk is hardly less august a role for a gay blade of a hero than to be a cockroach, if I may say so, and who among us can be unaware of the literary worth, the symbolic dimensions, of a cockroach?

Don't you think this story is coming along nicely? It is being written in a little house in the woods, before a stately mullioned window, as I eat a tuna fish sandwich, unfortunately garnished with pickle. The servant girl at this establishment, a saucy, charming young thing with fetching carroty hair, is all too fond of pickles. Out of mere indolence I suffer rather than complain. Outside, a badger shuffles aimlessly about the ashy trunk of a birch tree. I might even desert my desk and hyperpickled lunch to join him, for as our hero wrote at an advanced stage of wisdom, it is "just as fine a thing to be human and go for a walk as to sit at one's desk and successfully turn out books."

After his perky day of clerkiness, Walser would stop in a local café and drink his glass of beer with his fellow clerks and upright citizens, eyes somewhat glazed from the glare of their ruled ledgers. He might smoke a cigarette, for he was very attached to his cigarettes, a symptom not uncommon in clerks of the modern age. "I know a brand of cigarettes that lets me play the grand seigneur and smell terrific," he remarked. "Yesterday, by the way, I went a whole afternoon without smoking: an exercise in renunciation. People who can't renounce things never get to know the deeper pleasures."

A cigarette is a curious object, a heap of weeds rolled cylindrically into a paper and set on fire at one end. All manner of people put it to their lips, virtually kissing it with ardor, to draw in the fumes. A foul-smelling habit, certainly, yet one that has left an indelible, possibly salutary, mark on civilization. If not for the cigarette to quiet the nervous nerves, who knows how many more murders and acts of mayhem might have been perpetrated on suffering humanity? What might one not write about the effects of cigarettes on human history? And the effects of their renunciation as well, for now, the pundits tell us, these sweet weeds are unhealthy poisons. Yet away in the lands of the spicy East, potentates and peasants alike indulge in this fumy, curly, nasty habit, and seem none the worse. We must die of something, evidently. And a good thing too. Wouldn't you agree?

After his glass of beer, or his several beloved glasses of the sparkly, inspiriting brew, our little clerk—little not in size but in worldly position—would return to his cell, I mean, his room, to sit at another desk.

For, yes, there can be no more evading the subject: he was a clerk of another sort. He wrote: voluminously, incessantly, frivolously, profoundly, insanely, merrily, ambitiously, hopelessly. He wrote, he mailed his writings, though on occasion was known to burn them. Was he unhappy, you may well ask, when the mighty and learned editors of newspapers flew his pages back to him on billows of wind like flocks of paper airplanes? Unhappy because he was eternally poor and unrecognized? No, he was not unhappy. It would take more than such a mite to make our noble hero unhappy. "The apathy of an unappreciative public," he wrote, "will never do me in." He was ever cheerful and fun-loving, amusing the good townspeople with playful antics on his never-ending walks. And yet once in a while, perhaps he imagined himself unhappy. "It seems," he concluded as a young, or youngish man, "It seems one has only to imagine oneself unhappy to be so."

Still, for all his clerical fervor, our young man did not feel his deepest ambitions fulfilled. His taste for servility, that is to say, for knowledge, a prodigious, arrogant craving, was unsatisfied. Through forest and town he wended his way.

Woodland creatures cavorted in greeting. The tops of trees swayed at his approach. Streets crackled and blistered with excitement. And what a high old time he had. Through the great metropoli of Switzerland and Germany, through the highfalutin salons of the literary and artistic he strolled. He shook hands, now and then, with the great.

One glistening morning he approached the gates of a famous castle, guarded by customarily fierce men-at-arms, spears raised, visors lowered. Young Walser had to plunge through a perilous moat to reach its portals, thereby arriving at his destination in a fairly wettish condition. Nevertheless he was received, taken in, welcomed, embraced, in short, hired as butler. He served a mere three months, but ah, in those three months he served enough to last a lifetime. What did he not learn about the habits of the aristocracy at work and at play? About how to dust the statues of heroes of myth in a high-ceilinged salon, grovel to the steward and carry steaming soup to the table? But as with all things, his service came to an end. Back to the city, to the desk.

How he lived is something of a mystery. Isn't there a mystery to all lives, come to think of it? Isn't the shape of a life a question mark, with its initial optimistic curve, its gradual descent, and its diffident little point at the bottom, nodding farewell? Didn't our hero love questions? "Questions are usually more beautiful," he said, "more significant than their resolutions, which in fact never resolve them, are never sufficient to satisfy us, whereas from a question streams a wonderful fragrance."

They say he was like a child, so innocent and simple. But have you ever known an innocent, simple child who wrote a thousand and one hundred prose pieces? What did he think, our nominally childlike Walser, all those decades at the desk, rich in poverty, writing novels destined to feed his fireplace?

Did he wish he had married a lovely lady with bosom and bustle and plumed hat, one of the festooned ladies adorning the cafés, or possibly a brown-legged child of the forest, a woodland dryad living on nuts and berries? One way or the other, did he picture himself dandling a bunch of babbling babes on his knees? Oh, I don't know. People expect authors to know too much. I know he wrote, "The best thing will be to beget a child and offer the product to a publisher, who's hardly likely to reject it."

Do you think he longed for solace and recognition? I suppose he did. Who doesn't? Am I right or am I right? But he was an aimless sort of fellow, like my badger. Aimless, aimful. A cheery sort of melancholic fellow. "Aimlessness," he wrote in his wee, indecipherable script, upon a scrap of paper originally wrapping his bakery roll, "leads to the aim, while firm intentions often miss. When we strive too zealously, it may happen that our strivings harm us. I would advise speedy slowness or slow rapidity. Still, advice can't be more than advice." How abundantly correct, friend Walser of the buttonless waistcoat.

At last this fellow grew so melancholically confused that he was taken to the hospital by his sister, an upstanding lady whom I have woefully neglected in my story. Neglect is the literary fate, alas, of some quite worthy characters. He was examined, scrutinized, so to speak, by the holy priests, I mean the doctors. Did he want to go, you ask? Well, of course he did, unless he really didn't. He had a genius for bowing to the inevitable. "In renunciation of every sort," said he, "I became a great artist."

He went, and there he stayed, among the madmen whose words were as bizarre as pomegranates. I confess it embarrasses me—my face is all red; lucky no one can see me writing—to bring him to such a pass. I didn't want my story to wind up this way but what can a helpless author do? I wanted him to be a literary grandee, his name on the wet, greedy lips of posterical readers. A madman they called him, a madman he became. Or behaved, anyway. And with his gentle, serviceable temperament, even in the hospital he served—the doctors, that is, who always need to employ patients. Which is not to say he never smiled. As he was overheard to murmur, "There are moments, after all, when one feels compelled to smile although gripped with horror."

That is the last we hear from young Walser, nearly old by this time. His lips, as they say, were sealed, like a nun's body. And why did he not continue to write his frivolous, leafy, bucolic, terrifying little questioning, earnest, dissembling, skeptical, merry and artifactual prose pieces? Surely they would grant him pencil and paper, even in a hospital? Perhaps he had no more to say. Perhaps they convinced him he was nuts? "Trot, trot, trot," he wrote in his last prose piece, not really the last, only so called. "What's with me? Have I gone a bit nuts? What's going to become of me?"

Some say he was in despair, some say he was happy. I don't say anything at all. I hope you don't think this is unfair. I certainly wouldn't want to be thought unfair by anyone, most of all by a reader. I can tell you, since you clearly thirst for more information, that he said, "I think the best thing for me would be to sit in a corner and be quiet."

Silently he died in the snow, as foretold in the beginning. (Editors, please note the full circle!) Walking in the snow, painfully he parted company from this life. For as he once confided, "It is a very painful thing, having to part company with what torments you." Some children found him, as they gamboled on the slope with their dog. "Ho, ho, what's this, a melancholic genius-author lying in the snow?" they cried, and the dog barked, but Walser the friendly could not stroke him anymore. He could only lie in the embrace of the snow angel his body made as it fell.

Perhaps the children were horrified at the sight, or perhaps not; one never can tell with children. If they were, so much the better: "Why should horror not grip us modern people, slightly? It seems to me that we do very much need to be woken up, to be given a shake." In their horror or in the elation of discovery, the little ones ran off to alert their plump rosy mother, busy making a dinner of roast lamb and potatoes with succulent Brussels sprouts bathed in drippy butter, her face all asweat, her hair awry. The dinner, as you can guess, was late that night. Her husband, a sturdy bald farmer with a conspicuous wart on his left cheek, was considerably put out as a result. Marital disharmony ensued in the cottage after the children were put to bed. The mother shed a tear for the poor old man in the snow, for all mothers have tender hearts. So did the servant girl, or scullery maid as she was called, weep for him, a plain creature, I have been told, but with the most delicate white fingers and moonlike fingernails.

"Just one of those loonies from down the mountain," the farmer said, more harshly than he should. "Stop your sniveling and carry out the ashes." A boorish, heartless fellow who had never read a line of our illustrious hero's. No doubt if he had, he would have remembered. "At least we should learn to understand our fellow beings, for we are powerless to stop their misery, their ignominy, their suffering, their weakness and their death."

And the dog? Well, the dog just barked, musing silently—for he was an intelligent dog, a brown-and-white Saint Bernard who, unlike his crude master, had read a bit of Walserian prose in a newspaper long ago—"You and others expected much from the modern age. But it's not turning out quite the way you imagined."

The dead fellow was not to rest there in the snow, though, that glistening fresh mountain snow worshipped by skiers far and wide, its flakes settling like weary flowers on his brow. He was to be resurrected. And oh, patient readers, what the critics said of him! They could not bear to leave him a question mark. Their analyses and speculations are far beyond my gifts to recount. Our hero, the snow prince, could he read what they surmised of him, would laugh his melancholic laugh and say, "I was sparsely read, both at home and abroad, but even so there are people who think highly of me because of this."

And now what more to add? For when an author has taken her hero up to his death and even beyond it, surely she has reached the end of her little treatise, and may be granted surcease from sorrow. "Life, after all, writes such beautiful works. Isn't that enough for us?"

Three Walks on Corn Hill Beach

Corn Hill Beach, on the bay side of Cape Cod in Massachusetts, is not far from the tip of land where the narrowing, curving peninsula of the Upper Cape yields to water. You approach Corn Hill along a path of wooden boards partially covered with sand; you look up and suddenly it's there—shore, bay and sky—in all its understated brilliance, an oxymoron, yet it suits Corn Hill, so arresting yet so mild in character. To the north its shore sweeps a gentle arc toward Provincetown, whose notably phallic monument shows mistily in the distance, and to the south it stretches to the narrow harbor of the Pamet River hemmed in by seaweed-strewn dunes and jagged boulders where, bending over in the shallows, I once lost a pair of sunglasses. In the distance, nothing but sky, or the occasional Sunfish tilting in the wind. Its beauty is rivaled only by Long Nook Beach on the ocean side, whose high dunes cast giant shadows as the afternoon lowers.

I chose Corn Hill as the best place to walk away the hours of my brother's ordeal by a surgeon's knife till the phone call would come to relieve my mind, or not. Beyond its splendor, it was historically significant, not only publicly but privately. A plaque proclaimed it to be the spot where the Pilgrims first landed, although several other plaques on the Cape claim this distinction as well, so the Pilgrims seem to have made several stops. Its private history went back over forty years, to the summers we first came here with our small children and they found beach friends, instant intimacies that sprang up during the construction of forts and moats or hunting for hermit crabs to place in buckets of water where they flailed about, and ended abruptly when the parents were ready to go home.

I walked past the scattered blankets and umbrellas, to-day's children building their castles and moats in the mud. It was morning; there weren't yet many people about. I walked in the direction of the harbor and was soon alone, not far from the section set aside by the thinnest of cords, almost invisible, for the nesting terns, who with a touch of arrogance would spread their great wings to glide over the bay. Not like the plebeian seagulls, who wandered about picking at crumbs and bits of shells smelling of fish. Or the much smaller sandpipers, who appeared in late afternoon, hopping about like marionette birds controlled by strings.

I was trying to tire myself out until I was too tired to worry about my brother, so I walked all the way to the harbor, where I stood on the rocks and watched a few small boats pull in and be hoisted up to shore on a broad slanted gangplank. On the way back I stopped and sat on the sand. I had a sudden urge to swim. The water looked so inviting; it drew me powerfully. But I had no bathing suit; I hadn't planned to swim, only walk. I must have thought that bringing a bathing suit would denote a pleasure trip, while I was dedicating the hours to worrying. It seemed wrong, somehow, to set out for a swim while my brother was having his chest broken open. I was even faintly guilty about being away on vacation while he was lying on that table, but there was no help for that—he'd been stricken suddenly.

I wanted very badly to swim. I looked around; no one was in sight. I hesitated to take off my clothes and plunge in.

Lynne Sharon Schwartz

I dithered for a few moments till at last I thought, the hell with it, my brother is having his bare chest invaded, surely I can find the courage to take off my clothes. I stripped off my shorts and shirt and went in the water in nothing but bra and underpants. I felt very daring. I splashed around, swam a bit, floated on my back and watched the lazy clouds bump into each other. I was quite pleased at having done exactly what I wanted, casting aside inhibition.

I didn't rush out and, when I finally went ashore, didn't hurry to put on my clothes. I had to walk all the way back with my wet underwear under my shorts and shirt but this did not spoil my pleasure. If my brother had not survived, I might have felt guilty, but as it turned out, he did survive.

Several years later, I went again to Corn Hill to minister to my grief, a different kind of grief this time. (My brother was fine now, hale as before, and often when I phoned, he answered panting because he was running on the treadmill in his basement.) This time I didn't walk. I sat on the beach on a towel staring at the water but seeing the images I'd seen on television the night before in a bar, since my apartment had no TV. A friend I'd made in town and I had tickets to a play at the Provincetown Inn, a play about the relationship between Eleanor Roosevelt and her journalist friend and probably lover, Lorena Hickok. We didn't know what else to do with ourselves given the morning's attacks in New York under a dazzlingly blue sky, so we went to see the play, though we felt slightly uncomfortable, even oddly disloyal, doing so. The play was distracting, but as soon as it was over, our thoughts returned to the events in New York, and we went into a bar to see the images again.

As I sat on my towel staring at the images in my head, a man and a woman walked by in their bathing suits. The

176

woman was crying; her hands covered her face. The man had his arm around her shoulder. I understood her and felt just as she did, though I wasn't crying aloud and I didn't feel like walking, only sitting. And I was up here alone, not on a family vacation but working. I was staying in a small apartment in Provincetown for the month of September and used to drive to the beach when I judged I had done enough work for the day. Today I hadn't done any work at all, just made some phone calls, or tried to. The lines were mostly tied up. The automated voice kept saying try your call later.

It was afternoon now, high tide. The tides shift back and forth roughly every six hours. In other years, when I was here with my family, some days we'd stay at the beach long enough to watch the tide go out and see the sunset; or we'd return to Corn Hill at low tide to watch the sun sink into the bay like a huge cookie dipped very slowly into frosting. A crowd would gather in the evening as at a performance. The sun going down, however spectacular, was nothing strange, but the change in the bay was very strange indeed, though we had seen it happen many times. Where there had been water deep enough to swim in, there were mud flats, dotted with shells and small rocks, interspersed with shallow puddles. The setting sun glinted on the thin patina of water covering the mud, making it glow orange and gold. We could walk far out on the flats, maybe close to a quarter of a mile, much farther than we would have swum at high tide. Despite the tides' schedule of every six hours, more or less, for reasons I can't explain it was often at its lowest in the evening when the sun was setting.

There were people swimming that afternoon, though not as many as usual. Children clambered around on plastic tubes and giant plastic animals and others carried pails of sand back and forth from their building sites. But a curious hush hung over the beach, as if even the children were soft-ening their shouts out of respect for the thousands of dead, and there were fewer encampments of blankets and umbrel-las than usual, or fancy big tents in vivid colors, as if they hesitated to disrupt the general sobriety by their dazzle.

After a while I made myself get up and drive to the main pier in Provincetown to meet the ferry from Boston. My daughter would be on it. She was coming up to meet me and share the drive home to New York, because in my mood of shock and desolation I couldn't face the six-hour drive by myself. I parked and walked way out on the pier to where the boats docked. Many people were gathered, as always, to meet the ferry. They were in bright shirts and shorts and color-ful sleeveless dresses and they were tanned. We could see the ferry when it was still far out in the bay, then it rounded the breakwater and approached. It lumbered in, the gangplanks were lowered, and the passengers appeared, dragging their suitcases on wheels. I had witnessed this scene many times. People greeted their friends and relatives on the pier, falling into each other's arms. A few looked as stunned as I felt, as the woman on the beach had been, but most of them greeted each other gaily, as always when the ferry docked. I didn't look at them very closely, though; I was watching for my daughter. Finally she appeared, not dragging a suitcase but wearing a backpack. She would stay only a night or two and then we would go home.

Even from a distance her face looked as if it had been dipped in ashes. I studied some of the others from the fer-ry more closely and their faces had the same ashy look. My daughter gazed around at the scene—all the lively features of a summer resort—as if she had disembarked onto another planet. She said that after the hours in New York following the attack, the scene struck her as surreal—the people dressed like tropical birds, hugging and slapping each other's backs and hurrying off to their cars to begin a long beach weekend. She didn't want to talk much. We got in the car and drove to the apartment I was renting but would be leaving very soon. All I wanted was to be at home, closer to the rubble.

On another afternoon as I walked along the edge of the shore at Corn Hill (no shock or anxiety this time, just a pleasant beach day), I came upon a woman with a digital camera taking photos, or maybe a video, of her husband—I assumed it was her husband—and their three young children frolicking in the water. The woman was pretty far up on the sand and the man and children maybe a dozen feet off in the water, so to avoid being in the photo I would have had to diverge from my path and walk a broad arc around her. I didn't feel like doing that. I didn't know the etiquette for digital cameras—this was when they were new. Naturally if the photographer and her object had been only a few feet apart I would have walked politely around her; also, it struck me as odd to take a photo from so far off. So I walked in the path of the photography.

Somewhere, someday, when the woman shows her photos or video, a viewer will ask, Who's that?, meaning the woman in the black-and-white bathing suit going by. Oh, just someone passing on the beach, she'll say, and that will be all.

I will exist, or rather my image will exist, in their photo archives. That couple was much younger than I. In their archives my image, proof of my existence, will outlast me. Just a stranger passing by, with no history or identity beyond what can be seen from a distance in an amateur photo: a middle-aged woman, on the small side, dark curly hair, in a black-and-white one-piece bathing suit. A person who once existed and passed through their lives with no impact whatsoever (unless you count the interruption), and of no significance to them whatsoever. When I recall that moment or imagine that family, years from now, looking over old vacation photographs, I have a fleeting urge to let them know that I am—or was—something more than a stranger passing through their sight line, someone with a complete identity, whose life did have an impact on and significance for many others. Someone who had walked on that beach many times, usually reveling in its beauty, but on occasion dazed and grief-stricken. But of course that would be impossible, and moreover it's not a very strong urge. More of a mild notion, the way you don't especially care what will happen after you're dead, in regard to many things you care passionately about now.

Harmony

When I was eleven, I began a novel about twin girls. It was a crime novel: a body, a hotel room. I was fascinated by hotels though I had never stayed in one. To stay in a hotel seemed the pinnacle of glamour and sophistication. At that age, indeed well into adulthood, until I actually stayed in one, I dreamed of hotels. I longed to stay in a real hotel with a front desk and a lobby with armchairs and carpets and potted plants and uniformed bellhops.

Since it was not from experience, it was probably from the movies that I got the idea of what a hotel, a four- or five-star hotel, and its lobby should look like. The management would be visible and haughty and uniformed and the lobby active with guests yet serenely dignified, the kind of hotel a character in a 1940s movie would check into, where the bell-boy would follow in the elevator with the bags and lead the guest to a suite, fling open the windows and unobtrusively accept a tip. Then the guest would hurriedly make an important phone call or receive a visit from a mysterious stranger, or alternatively from some thugs sent to beat him up, and if the latter, he would awaken, dazed, send for Room Service and soon a wheeled tray would arrive with a bottle of champagne and a huge silver dome covering the meal; or if he never awakened from the beating, a maid in a white ruffled apron and cap would discover the body when she came in with a pile of towels and would start to scream. My novel would take place in a hotel like that.

I worked on the novel in the most dismal and unhotel-like of places, in school, in the seventh grade. The last class on Friday afternoon was reserved for Creative Arts. The week was almost over, so I suppose the authorities thought there was no harm in spending a smidgen of time on something as harmless as the arts—a dessert after the meat-and-potatoes subjects. Most of the class drew or did clay modeling but a few of us were permitted to sit at our desks and write. For forty-five minutes I would cover sheet after sheet of a yellow legal pad, flipping each one over in haste.

The plot turned on the twins being identical. One of them would die and the other would be left bereft, either to carry on her sister's life or to solve the mystery—I never figured out exactly where the story would go after the initial murder. The notion of twins, like that of hotels, was another of my secret fantasies. I never imagined I was adopted, or a changeling, as so many children do, but I did suspect I might be a twin. My thoughts would often unreel in dialogue, as if I were speaking to someone, a double, who would receive my words with perfect understanding. I had friends, but they knew me piecemeal; only this double could receive and thoroughly grasp everything about me. My thoughts and feelings, my doings, needed to be put into words and offered to this double for validation. Until then, they felt less than real, less than achieved. Only words—formulated and offered— could give my life the definitive stamp of reality.

So I spoke to her, my imagined twin, but it was I who contributed her half of the dialogue. This left me puzzled and uneasy. Where was she? I overheard that my mother had had several miscarriages and that one of those pregnancies was twins. It wasn't out of the question, then, that I, too, could be a twin and my double had died at birth. I imagined that my family had conspired to keep this secret from me, thinking it would distress me, but the uncertainty and puzzlement were even more distressing. The vanished twin would explain why I felt vaguely lonely and kept trying to talk to someone exactly like myself who would understand me effortlessly, and why she didn't answer. Later on I learned that some fetuses start out as twins but one embryo fails to develop; perhaps it emerges with the placenta or just melts away somehow. I cultivated the notion that I'd been half of such a pregnancy—this notion exonerated my family from being unduly secretive—and that it was my undeveloped, unborn double whom I kept trying to talk to. That must be why my early novel had twins as its main characters, and why one of them had to die.

I didn't finish that novel in the seventh grade. Either the term was over, or Creative Arts was abandoned, or I lost interest or didn't know how to proceed with the plot. From that effort, though, I grasped instinctively that writing was a place to indulge one's fantasies and try on costumes, to mask and multiply the self.

After I grew up, the story about the twins kept nagging at me. I moved around a lot and carried the idea with me, but was never able to make any headway. In the early years of my married life my husband got a Fulbright grant to study in Rome. While I was there, I tried to concentrate on writing, but I was not successful. All I could come up with were the beginnings of novels filled with violence and mayhem that led nowhere. It frightened me to think that I could harbor such violent fantasies, and so I would abandon them. Not a very professional attitude, but I was far, then from taking myself seriously as a writer, and from accepting my lurid fantasies with the equanimity I later acquired. Sometimes in desperation I thought of reviving that old mystery story about the twins and the hotel room that I'd started in the seventh grade, but I never got beyond thinking about it.

Years later, when I was teaching in Southern California and after I had written several other books, again I attempted that unfulfilled mystery begun in the seventh grade. Again it was about identical twins, and rather melodramatic. As before, one would die and the other live on, forever missing her sister. And again I found myself yearning for a double—a gifted writer—who perhaps could help out by providing a first draft. First drafts are always the most difficult part of writing, and I have always wished someone could do them for me. Afterward, I'd be more than happy to rewrite as much as necessary.

This time, even without an accommodating double, I did manage to write a good bit, but again never finished. I couldn't work out the plot, but even more, I couldn't work out what it all meant, what it was *for*. The story was a series of calamities befalling a family, but it had no underlying purpose. I think I simply enjoyed heaping tragedy at the doorstep of this unfortunate family, out of a masochistic anger that I had agreed to teach in Southern California, alone and alienated. Evenings I would eat dinner in front of the TV news. It was 1991. I watched the Gulf War—missiles exploding in air like a fireworks display, the commentators insanely gleeful about the new technology—and I watched the Los Angeles police beating Rodney King with their clubs, a scene shown every evening for weeks. After dinner and the war and the beating, I read. My stint in Southern California was ten weeks, so I was reading the longest novel I could find, Alessandro Manzoni's *The Betrothed*, which vividly depicted the fourteenth-century plague. Decaying, pustulating bodies lay crammed together in smelly shelters, while two forcibly separated lovers searched for each other. No wonder I took out my frustrations on that poor family I invented.

For a long time after that, I carried those melodramatic pages with me—one twin doomed in adolescence, the other doomed to live bereft—wherever I went, but couldn't make anything coherent out of them. Meanwhile, I kept writing other books.

Very soon after the September 11 attacks on the World Trade Center, I enrolled in an evening course in Harmony. I'd started picking out tunes on the piano when I was four or five years old, and at six I began taking lessons. Even though I took piano lessons for thirteen years and became a fairly decent amateur pianist, and even though I went diligently through all the scales, chords, and arpeggios, I never achieved a coherent understanding of theory and harmony. For years I mused on and off about remedying this lack and even tried on my own with books, but had little success.

The attack itself was so arresting and unanticipated that I could barely think about anything else. Writing felt impossible. The event was a boulder in my mind that I couldn't get past. That entire autumn, the downtown site was all everyone in New York thought about and talked about. A half mile north, you could see thin curls of smoke still rising, slow and reluctant. When I closed my eyes, the iconic images of the towers falling and the debris lined the insides of my lids. The newspapers were filled with stories of the dead, new and unforgettable gory details coming to light daily, alongside the dense, specious language of political and military maneuvering.

One night, as I was leafing through a brochure of concerts and courses offered by a local music school, my eye caught a description of the Harmony course. The next minute I was filling out a form in the back of the brochure. I suppose I wanted to fix my attention, if only for two hours a week, on a subject as far as possible from downtown Manhattan. That must have been why I chose that moment, of all the moments since I stopped taking piano lessons, to become a student of Harmony.

The class was held in a building near Lincoln Center that in the daytime served as a public elementary school for children gifted in music. Our room was a first-grade classroom, not too different from the seventh-grade classroom in which I had begun my mystery novel about the twins, but everything was on a smaller scale, befitting younger children. The walls were lined with the letters of the alphabet in capital and lowercase, as well as with pictures of animals, their names printed below in that clear typeface used for small children. There were children's drawings hanging on the walls too. In the midst of the mourning outside those walls, the downtown air thick with the smell of smoke bearing the traces of charred flesh, it was soothing to gaze at crayoned pictures of A-frame houses with curling smoke—innocent smoke—wafting from squat chimneys, of daisies and horses and tricycles, trucks and dogs and oceans made of parallel wavy lines.

We didn't sit in the tiny first-grade chairs—they were stacked up against a wall while we used metal folding chairs—yet there was a sense of miniaturization about the class. Everything, including the room itself, was small and enclosed and manageable. At the front, to one side, was an old upright piano. Facing us was an old-fashioned blackboard. Three horizontal rows of chairs were set up, six chairs in each row, but they were not filled. The class had about eight or ten students, but some nights only five or six attended. I never missed a class. It was the happiest time of my week; I looked forward to it.

The teacher was a very animated, slight, good-looking mustached man named Victor, around forty or so. On the first night Victor instructed us to go out and buy a small music notebook, which I duly did, and I took it to class each week, along with pencils with good erasers, feeling that I was back in elementary school, though I enjoyed the Harmony class more than I had ever enjoyed elementary or any other school, far more than I had enjoyed the seventh grade, despite the bonus of Creative Arts.

Victor was an ideal teacher. He always arrived promptly. He shimmered with energy and taught with enthusiasm. He moved swiftly and wrote swiftly on the blackboard, his rendering of the notes possessing a dashing grace quite different from my clumsy, childish efforts. He began the course with the most fundamental aspects of theory: the major and minor scales, the chords, the intervals, all of which were familiar to me, but I didn't mind the repetition. I had learned it piecemeal, not in any orderly fashion. Now I loved the way everything fit into a stable and superbly logical whole. Victor progressed weekly from the simple to the more complex, making everything clear and manageable. He taught us about the circle of fifths—the major and minor scales arranged in a perfect circle, a rational, balanced miniature universe—and he made it so clear that I thought I could never forget it. But I have forgotten it, mostly.

Along with the technical material, Victor regaled the class with savory anecdotes about music, musicians, and amusing moments and milestones in the history and development of harmony, and I took copious notes in my little notebook. As he spoke, in his witty and animated way, about the intricacies and subtleties and private jokes of harmony, it seemed there was nothing else of importance in the world except this subject, Harmony, which was of surpassing, crucial importance. For those two hours, my attention was heartfelt and thorough. Everything outside was forgotten; it was as if the attacks had never happened. Only Harmony existed.

In school I had never been one of those students who crowd around the teacher after class, yet here I often stayed a few extra minutes to ask Victor questions. These were not merely pretexts to prolong the respite, however. I had serious and pressing questions about harmony and felt I could not go home unless my curiosity was satisfied. Today I remember none of these questions or their answers.

Each week he gave us homework. We had to devise simple harmonies—eight or so bars of music—for four voices, bass, tenor, alto and soprano, which meant making up four little tunes that fit together according to the principles of harmony. I enjoyed doing my homework—above all the very idea of homework—and would usually do it as soon as I got home after class, so I wouldn't forget the points in the lesson that needed to be incorporated in the homework. Each week Victor would put one person's homework assignment on the blackboard and we would analyze it to see how well it conformed to the principles of harmony. The night he asked for my assignment I was quite excited. I tore it out of my notebook and handed it to him with a flourish, which made him laugh. He dissected my homework, and though it contained a few small infelicities, overall it was fairly successful, and I was as proud as if I were in first grade and had read aloud, to near-perfection, a passage from a Dick and Jane primer.

As the term drew to a close, he suggested that we might want to take the next course in the series on harmony, in which the homework would no doubt be more complicated. I considered taking this course but never did.

I no longer remember any of the other students, yet I think of them, vague warm bodies in the seats around me, as my companions during that awful time when, outside of Tuesday night's Harmony class, the city was grieving and awash in confusion. I still have my little notebook with all my homework assignments and class notes—the one assignment I ripped out to hand to Victor sticking out with its jagged edge. I look at it sometimes, without opening it, and am reminded of that oasis of harmony, Tuesday nights at six-fifteen, moving from the luminous blue-skied autumn into the cold winter of resignation, through the various kinds of intervals, and always the perfect foundation of the circle of fifths, while outside the little room came anthrax and Afghanistan and the daily funerals and the recovery of body parts.

When the course was over, the world outside still remained, and what was I to do about it? I thought maybe it was time to write something again. If I stop writing even for a couple of weeks, I worry that I'm not really a writer anymore, and that feeling returned in force. I would have to write something about what had just happened in New York City because it was still a boulder in my mind and nothing else could get past it. But where to begin? Once again I remembered those old pages in my desk drawer about the doomed twins from the family on whom, in my loneliness and frustration in Southern California, I had heaped tragedy, a tragedy that hadn't added up to anything useful in a literary sense.

I took out those old pages, and in this new context of the terrorist attacks, they made sense. At least I saw a way they could begin to cohere. As before, one twin would die early on, and the remaining twin's grief would be evoked later on as a memory. But the story of her life would have to be redesigned, for along with the private tragedy would be added the greater, public tragedy, the two permeating each other. The narrative would no longer be an assemblage of pointless mayhem, but could take a useful place in the larger world, as an attempt to make a pattern out of what had happened. It would have the context and the purpose it had lacked before. Instead of creeping around the boulder in my mind, I would drill my way through it.

So at last I was able to finish my story about the twins. It was as if my story had been waiting all along for its meaning. I jettisoned the hotel setting. By that time I had stayed in many hotels and was no longer awed by their glamour. But more important, in this new context, hotels no longer mattered. They were like the crumpled-up newspaper that you use to set a good log fire and that disappears in the blaze of its own making. Far more significant than hotels were communal grief and shock and their aftermath, the need to undergo and assimilate them. Those would be the core of the story I began at eleven years old in the seventh grade on Friday afternoons at two-fifteen in Creative Arts, decades before anyone ever dreamed that the World Trade Center would be built, still less that it would be destroyed one sunny autumn morning.

"A Refreshing Change

Is in Your Future"

In March of 2020 when the pandemic threatened and the lockdown began, I thought of all the spare time I would have. New Yorkers love to boast about how busy they are, a dubious point of pride. Among friends, subtle competitions can simmer: Busier Than Thou. Now, with everyone working from home or out of work, a peculiar unease arose: instead of having no spare time, could we have too much?

I had just completed writing a book and wasn't ready to start another. My teaching job, now online, was part-time. Acres of time unfurled before me—what I had always longed for—yet I found myself slightly alarmed at the prospect. No work deadlines, no visits with friends, no theaters or movies, no museums. Even my weekly volunteer work was canceled. There was always walking and reading, but ... what else would I do?

Obviously this was the moment to start projects there'd never been enough time for, and I don't mean cleaning out closets. (One of my daughters once remarked that whenever I finish a book, I start cleaning closets.) But I wanted to use the time in a more productive, or at any rate enjoyable, way.

I have absolutely no talent for the visual arts, nor had I ever ventured to learn. Everything I knew how to do was connected to music (piano and West African drums) or to language— reading, writing, translating. All my life, I realized with creep-

Lynne Sharon Schwartz

ing dismay, I had stuck to those and avoided learning anything unfamiliar, anything that did not come naturally. Even in college, I had contrived to take only the minimum of required courses in other areas. In a manner of speaking I had never learned anything new, that is, anything that would train my mind to move along new pathways.

There was one thing I had always had a yen to do, though, and that was make collages. Surely anyone, even without artistic talent, could cut and paste. And I had a fairly good eye: I could tell original from banal, pleasing from clumsy. Not that what I made needed to be original or even pleasing. Unlike with writing, I was not seeking an audience. What better time?

I dug up a shopping bag full of scraps of leftover wrapping paper, which I'd been saving for when I had free time. I bought some large poster board and glue sticks, spread newspapers over the dining room table and got to work. My first effort was meant to represent the painful experiences of immigrants at the border crossings in Texas, an awful situation that was getting worse. From some old Christmas wrapping paper I cut out figures of children; from colored construction paper I made a long wavy blue strip to represent a river, and a bland beige shape to represent the desert. These and more were pasted on varied shapes of more colored paper. The finished product had no artistic value whatsoever and probably couldn't be understood, but I'd loved doing it. I showed it to my family, like a child proudly bringing home a kindergarten project, and while they were kind, they were puzzled. To make my theme absolutely clear, I added words in caps: RIVER; DESERT; FENCE; BORDER GUARDS. I sprinkled the whole thing with letters that spelled CRUELTY.

So even my "artwork" couldn't escape words altogether. My powers of visual expression weren't enough. Then I remembered my large collection of Chinese fortune cookie sayings, which I'd been saving for years. I loved the amusing cliches that everyone reads after dinner in a Chinese restaurant. ("You are soon going to change your present line of work.")

I decided to assemble a large collage of my collection, with the fortunes pasted onto colorful backgrounds. To start, I typed them all into a document and chose a different typeface for each one, enlarged enough to be readable from a few feet away. I was amazed at the dozens of exotic fonts my computer offered; if I ever wrote anything again, I thought I could use them to liven up my manuscript.

I cut them all out and cut out a bunch of oddly shaped backgrounds of construction paper, then painstakingly assembled the whole work. ("Any job, big or small, do it right or not at all.") I wanted a haphazard look, which it definitely had: no familiar geometrical shapes, no discernible order, just cheerful chaos—a freedom I could never exercise in writing or music, where I knew too much. In this field I knew nothing, no tradition to aspire to, no models to emulate. No public would see or judge them. I knew great artists had made collages, but those were so remote from my efforts that I didn't even consider them. ("Never compare yourself to the best others can do, but to the best you can do.") I could do whatever I wanted. I was thrilled with the result. It turned out that over years of Chinese meals I had collected too many fortunes to fit on one 3-by-4-foot board, so I went through the whole process again.

Now I have the two posters decorating the walls of my study, and when I look up from my desk, I can take courage from "Focus on the main task at hand" or "You are offered the dream of a lifetime. Say yes!" But there was one that I disobeyed: "Depart not from the path which fate has you assigned." At long last, I had departed from the path that fate assigned me. I tried something I had no innate aptitude for. I learned what it is to learn.

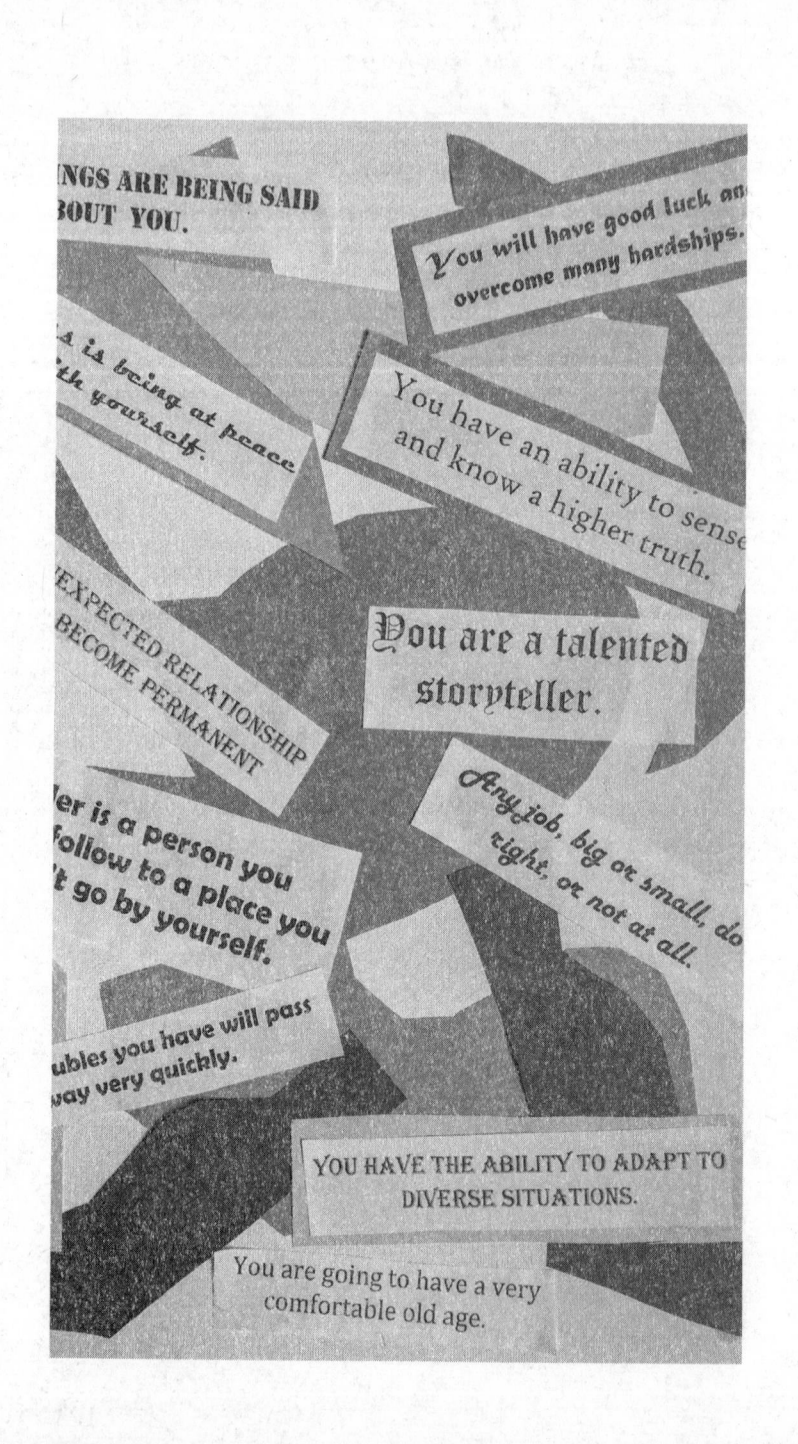

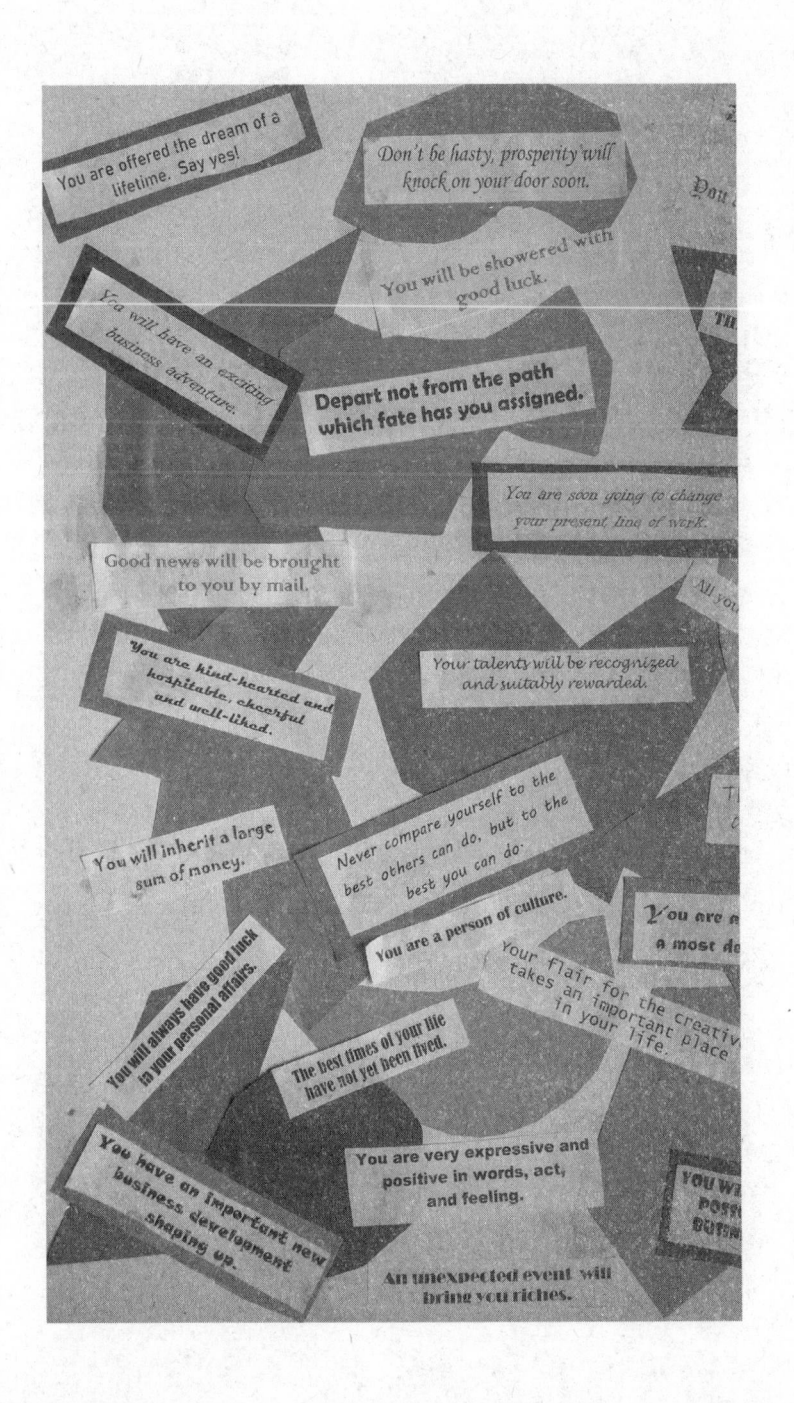

Acknowledgments

"You Gotta Have Heart"—*Agni*, shorter version; my essay collection, *This Is Where We Came In*

"My Mother Speaks,"—*I've Always Wanted to Tell You, Letters to Our Mothers*, ed. Constance Warloe

"The Renaissance"—*Brief Encounters*, anthology ed. Dinah Lenney and Judith Kitchen

"Degrees of Separation"—*Literal Latte*

"What I Don't Know"—*The American Scholar, online*

"The Other Henry James"—*Threepenny Review*

"Using a Cane"—*The American Scholar*

"First Loves"—My poetry collection, *No Way Out But Through*

"Beyond the Garden"—*Belles Letters*

"Only Connect"—*Salmagundi*, short version; *Tolstoy's Dictaphone*, anthology ed. Sven Birkerts

"Give Me Your Tired, Your Poor . . ."—*The American Scholar*

"Time Off to Translate"—Under the title, "Found in Translation," *American Literary Review*, and my book of essays, *Face to Face*

"Detective Briscoe of the NYPD"—*New York Times* City Section

"A Sort of Hero"—*Review of Contemporary Fiction*

"Harmony"—*Northwest Review*

"A Refreshing Change Is in Your Future"—*The American Scholar*, online

About the Author

Lynne Sharon Schwartz is the author of twenty-eight books of fiction, essays, and poetry, including her 2021 story collection, *Truthtelling*, as well as the novels *Disturbances in the Field*, *Leaving Brooklyn*, a finalist for the PEN/Faulkner Award, and *Rough Strife*, a finalist for the National Book Award. She has also published two memoirs, *Ruined by Reading* and *Not Now, Voyager*, and has translated from the Italian. Schwartz is the recipient of fellowships from the Guggenheim Foundation, the National Endowment for the Arts in Fiction and, separately, for Translation, and the New York State Foundation for the Arts Fellowship. She has taught widely in the United States and abroad, most recently at the Bennington College Writing Seminars and the Columbia University School of the Arts.